W0090499

Pharmacy Administration

GVRK Acharyulu

Faculty Member
School of Management Studies
University of Hyderabad
Hyderabad

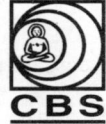

CBS

CBS Publishers & Distributors Pvt Ltd

New Delhi • Bengaluru • Chennai • Kochi • Kolkata • Mumbai
Hyderabad • Nagpur • Patna • Pune • Vijayawada

Disclaimer

Science and technology are constantly changing fiel
New research and experience broaden the scope
information and knowledge. The author has tried
best in giving information available to him wh
preparing the material for this book. Although, all effc
have been made to ensure optimum accuracy of tl
material, yet it is quite possible some errors might ha
been left uncorrected. The publisher, the printer ar
the author will not be held responsible for a
inadvertent errors, omissions or inaccuracies.

Pharmacy Administration

ISBN: 978-81-239-2580-6

Copyright © Author and Publisher

CBS Reprint: 2015

Reprint: 2016 , 2019

All rights reserved. No part of this book may be reproduced or transmitted in any form or by any means, electronic or mechanical, including photocopying, recording, or any information storage and retrieval system without permission, in writing, from the author and the publisher.

Published by Satish Kumar Jain and produced by Varun Jain for

CBS Publishers & Distributors Pvt Ltd

4819/XI Prahlad Street, 24 Ansari Road, Daryaganj, New Delhi 110 002, India.
Ph: 23289259, 23266861, 23266867   Website: www.cbspd.com
Fax: 011-23243014   e-mail: delhi@cbspd.com; cbspubs@airtelmail.in.

Corporate Office: 204 FIE, Industrial Area, Patparganj, Delhi 110 092
Ph: 4934 4934   Fax: 4934 4935   e-mail: publishing@cbspd.com; publicity@cbspd.com

Branches

- **Bengaluru:** Seema House 2975, 17th Cross, K.R. Road,
  Banasankari 2nd Stage, Bengaluru 560 070, Karnataka
  Ph: +91-80-26771678/79   Fax: +91-80-26771680   e-mail: bangalore@cbspd.com
- **Chennai:** 7, Subbaraya Street, Shenoy Nagar, Chennai 600 030, Tamil Nadu
  Ph: +91-44-26680620, 26681266   Fax: +91-44-42032115   e-mail: chennai@cbspd.com
- **Kochi:** Ashana House, No. 39/1904, AM Thomas Road, Valanjambalam,
  Eranakulam 682 018, Kochi Kerala
  Ph: +91-484-4059061-65   Fax: +91-484-4059065   e-mail: kochi@cbspd.com
- **Kolkata:** 6/B, Ground Floor, Rameswar Shaw Road, Kolkata-700 014, West Bengal
  Ph: +91-33-22891126, 22891127, 22891128   e-mail: kolkata@cbspd.com
- **Mumbai:** 83-C, Dr E Moses Road, Worli, Mumbai-400018, Maharashtra
  Ph: +91-22-24902340/41   Fax: +91-22-24902342   e-mail: mumbai@cbspd.com

Representatives

- **Hyderabad** 0-9885175004   • **Nagpur**   0-9021734563   • **Patna**   0-9334159340
- **Pune**   0-9623451994   • **Vijayawada** 0-9000660880

Printed at Swastik Packaging

Acknowledgements

This book would not have been possible without the support and help of many people who have provided us information and suggestions on various aspects. I acknowledge all of them.

I am are very thankful to Dr.B.Raja Shekhar, Associate Professor, School of Management Studies, University of Hyderabad for his encouragement and valuable suggestions from time to time in successfully finishing this text book. I also thank Mr. M. Sudhakar, Research Scholar, for his continuous support. .

I am thankful to my family members for their unconditional support and encouragement to pursue our interests.

I am very grateful to Ikon books for their cooperation in bringing out this volume.

I welcome comments and suggestions from users of this edition and I will highly appreciate them if they give me feed back to refine and improve this book in accordance with the changes and context in future.

Dr G V R K ACHARYULU

SEPTEMBER 2009

PREFACE

During last decade pharma industry under went a complete transformation due to liberalisation, globalisation, emerging GATT era and then India becoming a member of WTO coupled with major shift in Government's economic policy. All these events led to severe competition, demand of high quality standards of drugs and pharmaceuticals introduction of new generation of drugs, emerging biotechnological methods for the production of extremely efficacious drugs. Increased understandings of pattern of diseases due to advances in biology, immunology and microbiology have lead to the development of ultra sensive rapid diagnostic aids and tools. Along with these the availability of sophisticated biomedical equipments and instruments for diagnosis and new technologies and devices for the effective treatment of diseases. Such rapid advances demands the greater responsibility of pharmacists working in hospitals and community.

The pharmaceutical industries are already driven to adopt new corporate strategies, renewed management culture and systems, application of innovative technologies, intellectual related activities like Contract Clinical and developmental research, IPR, horizontal and vertical technology transfer, contract/toll manufacturing and marketing for their sustained growth and the very survival.

As the Indian pharmaceutical industry is growing rapidly with advent of technological developments, opening up of retail pharmacy chains, clinical research trials and new drug development, Pharmacy Administration has become vital to face the challenges in the healthcare industry.

Pharmacy Administration is a dynamic field that applies approaches from management science, economics, and the social sciences, to issues in healthcare that relate to pharmacy, pharmacists, and pharmaceuticals. Pharmacy administration deals with the business and managerial aspects of pharmacy in its broadest sense.

Pharmacy administration gives thrust on pharmaceutical products and service, pharmaceutical policy; medication compliance; rational drug use; drug distribution; socioeconomic and cultural issues related to drug use; evaluate health care intervention in terms of economic, humanistic and clinical outcomes; pharmacist-patient communications, and the role of pharmacist in managed care.

Pharmacy administration focuses on managing the financial, physical, and human resources involved in the practice of pharmacy and the healthcare industry. This course is to evaluate outcomes associated with pharmacy practice and drug utilization, resulting in optimal patient care.

Pharmacy administration enables pharmacists who have the abilities and skills which are necessary to achieve outcomes related to:

i). Providing pharmaceutical care to patients,

ii). Developing and managing medication distribution and control systems

iii). Managing the pharmacy

iv). Promoting public and private health

v). Providing drug information and education

The delivery of effective pharmaceutical care to patients requires pharmacists to practice in a way that uses their time effectively and reflects their responsibility and accountability. Ideally all patients who receive pharmaceutical products or services should also receive pharmaceutical care. Pharmacists stand at the interface between research and development, manufacturer, prescriber, patient and the medicine itself. The emerging trend is to develop new patient-oriented pharmaceutical care practices and thus to enhance the value of pharmacists in drug therapy management for the integration of pharmacists into the mainstream of service provision to physicians and patients.

The objective pharmacy administration is to develop administrative, managerial, marketing or pharmacoeconomic skills in the pharmaceutical industry, pharmacy education government agencies, health care institutions, community pharmacies, and pharmacy organizations.

Need for Pharmacy Administration:

i). Paper based prescription some times leads to medication errors

ii). Difficulty in managing drug inventory

iii). Needs to keep track of drugs expired

iv). Unavailability of medicine leads to loss of customers

v). Lack of database about new drug releases

vi). Lack of information to guide patients to various blood banks and organ banks

vii). Lack of information about near-by hospitals and other medical services

Every sphere of human activity now-a-days required management skills. The profession of pharmacy is no exception to this golden rule. As there is a tremendous growth of pharmaceutical industries in India, managers are likely to play a pro vital role in near future. It is important that the pharmacy administration will enable to gain knowledge of management principle and accountancy for judicious utilization of men, money and material in fulfilling the organizational goal and objectives.

In the light of the above, the entire book is divided into eight units. The first unit introduces introduction to Business and Organisation. Subsequently topics like characteristics organisation, types and business environment in post liberalisation scenario are dealt.

The second unit familiarizes the students with the concept of Manufacturing Management and aims at giving an overall picture production, plant location, layouts and new product development.

In the third unit, first part deals with Work study fundamentals and Quality concepts. The second part deals with Statistical Quality Control (SQC), acceptance sampling and Deming's contribution to quality.

The fourth unit is aimed at teaching the students about the Marketing concepts and organisation of distribution. The important aspects like marketing mix, marketing strategies based on Product Life Cycle (PLC) and sales promotion are discussed.

The fifth unit deals with growth of pharma industry covering structure, export and import trade of pharmaceuticals.

The sixth and seventh units focus on Types of Insurance including marine and health insurance. Subsequently the thrust is given on governance in pharmacy which consists of Pharmaceutical associations& societies and medical detailing

The last unit covers drug store planning, salesmanship, community pharmacy and accounting records.

This book gives a through knowledge on Pharmacy Administration to the students and for any further improvements do write to me.

Dr. G.V.R. K. Acharyulu

Table of Contents

Chapter - 8
Principles of drug store and community pharmacy administration

Chapter 1

FEATURES OF BUSINESS ORGANISATIONS & NEW ECONOMIC ENVIRONMENT

1.1 INTRODUCTION TO BUSINESS

A business may be defined as an institution organized and operated to provide goods and services to the society with the objective of earning profit. L.R. Dickson has defined business as a form of activity pursued primarily with the object of earning profit for the benefit of those on whose behalf the activity is conducted. "Business involves production and/or exchange of goods and services to earn profits or in a broader sense, to earn a living. Profit is not the sole objective of the business. It may have other objectives like promotion of welfare of the workers and the general public. Business activities include production and distribution of goods and services which can satisfy human wants.

The term business should be used to convey the same meaning as the term trade simply denotes purchase and sale of goods whereas 'business' includes all activities form production to distribution of goods and services. It embraces industry, trade and other activities like banking, transport, Insurance and warehousing which facilitates production and distribution of goods and services. According to F.C. Hopper "The whole complex field of commerce and industry which includes the basic industries, processing and manufacturing industries, and the network of ancillary services: distribution, banking, insurance transport and so on, which serve and inter penetrate the world of business as a whole" are called business activities.

Nature of Business

A business enterprise has the following characteristics:

1. **Dealing in Goods and Services :** The first basic characteristic of a business is that it deals in goods and services. Goods produced or exchanged may be consumer goods such as bread, rice, cloth, etc., or capital goods such as machines, tools, etc.,

The consumer goods are meant for direct consumption either immediately or after undergoing some processes, whereas the capital goods are meant for being used for the purpose of further production. Capital goods are also known as producer's goods. Services include supply of electricity, gas, water and finance, insurance, transportation, warehousing, etc.

2. **Production and Exchange:** Every business is concerned with production and exchange of goods and services for value (prices). Thus, goods produced or purchased for personal consumption (or) for presenting to others as gifts do not constitute business because there is no sale or transfer for value involved. If, for example 'A' buys a T.V. Set in Tokyo to be gifted to his brother on his return to New Delhi, it will not amount to business. But if the same person realize the price of the T.V. Set, it will come under the scope of business in a limited way provided the other conditions are also satisfied which are given below.

3. **Regularity and Continuity in Dealings:** One sale transaction cannot strictly constitute a business. A sale of a product can be called a business if it is undertaken frequently. If other essential characteristics of business are present and the production of goods or rendering of services for a price is undertaken regularly and continuously, this activity will be called a business.

4. **Uncertainty or Risk:** Business activities, as we have formed some definite ideas about it by now, carry an element of uncertainty or risk. It is true that the element of risk is present in almost all economic activities in a small or great measure. But it is certainly more significantly present in business activities. Risk involves the possibility of loss or what may be called uncertainty of return on investment made in the business due to a variety of factors over which the business enterprise has practically no control.

5. **Profit Motive:** Human-beings are engaged in business primarily with a view to earn profits and acquire wealth. This is not in any way reduce the importance of service motive in business. As a matter of fact, there is a positive relationship between proper and satisfactory services to the customers and to the society and the extent of profit. Normally, better services are accompanied by higher profits, but it may not always be so. Profit motive is also accepted as a desirable objective even for the Government enterprises engaged in business. It is called surplus instead of Profit in case of Government enterprises.

1.2 FUNCTIONS OF BUSINESS

In order to achieve its objectives, a business enterprise performs many functions which may be broadly grouped under the following headings: Production, Marketing, Finance and Personnel. In big business organisations, there are separate departments to look after these functional areas. It may be noted that these functions are interdependent and inter-related. For instance, production department depends upon marketing department to sell its output and marketing departments depends upon production department for the products of required quality to satisfy its customers. Thus, there must be proper integration of various functional areas of business to achieve its objectives. This can be achieved by the management of the enterprise by effective planning, organization, direction and control. The important functions of a business are briefly discussed below.

1. **Production Function:** It is concerned with the transformation of inputs like manpower, materials, machinery, capital, information and energy into specified outputs as demanded by the society. The production department is entrusted with so many activities such as production planning and control, quality control, procurement of materials and storage of materials.

2. **Marketing Function:** It is concerned with distribution of goods and services produced by the production department. It can perform this function efficiently only if it is able to satisfy the needs of the customers. For this purpose, the marketing department guides the production department in product planning and development. It fixes the prices of various products produced by the business. It promotes the sale of goods through advertisement and sales promotion devices such as distribution of samples and novelty items, holding contests, organizing displays and exhibitions, etc.

3. **Finance Function :** It deals with arrangement of sufficient capital for the smooth running of business. It also tries to ensure that there is proper utilization of resources. It takes many important decisions such as sources of finance, investment of funds in productive ventures, and levels of inventory of various items.

4. **Personnel Function :** This function is concerned with finding suitable employees, giving them training, fixing their remuneration and motivating them. The quality of human resource working in the enterprise is a critical factor in the achievement of business objectives. Therefore it is necessary that the work force is highly motivated and satisfied with the terms and conditions of service offered by the enterprise.

WHAT IS AN ORGANIZATION?

When two or more people get together and agree to coordinate their activities in order to achieve their common goals, an organization has been born. Its purpose is to create an arrangement of positions and responsibilities through and by means of which an enterprise can carry out its work.

An academic textbook definition of organization can be formulated as follows: "a. the responsibilities by means of which the activities of the enterprise are dispersed among the (managerial, supervisory, and specialist) personnel employed in its service; and b. the formal interrelations established among the personnel by virtue of such responsibilities."

It must be emphasized that an organization should not be seen as rigid as the term "framework" implies. In reality, almost all organization structures must be occasionally reviewed due to various changes in the external environment of the organization in question. Moreover, internal changes also occur oftentimes due to the development of various informal relationships. Few examples for organization are hospitals, colleges, factories, farms and government offices.

Organizational structure is the way in which the different groups of people, working in the organization, are constructed the objective of creating these groups are created to ensure proper coordination, less wastage of resources and quick achievement of objectives. These structures than take different forms like bureaucratic, functional structure, matrix structure, and divisional structures etc each structure has its own advantages. The shape adopted by a structure depends upon factors like the size of the organization, variety of operations being performed by the organization, number of branches and their location, education level of manpower, available resources

BUSINESS ORGANISATION:

Business organisation is a process or an art of establish effective cooperation between the factors of production (land, material, capital equipment, personnel) for producing or acquiring wealth with a view to earn profit in an enterprise.

The scope of business organization has considerably expanded after the industrial revolution. The process of production is now quite complicated. An organization is needed to determine what each person will do and how much authority each will have. We generally divided the organization into three forms on behave on business ownership; these forms are sole proprietorship, partnership and company.

Organization helps in the efficient use of factors of production and thus reduces cost of production of goods. This helps to attain the goals and objectives of the business at the minimum cost. A good organization provides for the optimum use of technological improvement to create goodwill. All the marketing functions of goods such as buying, selling, transportation, storage, financing, risk taking product standardization and grading, etc are solved by the organization by fixing of responsibilities to every one

Business organisation refers to all necessary arrangements required to conduct a business. It refers to all those steps that need to be undertaken for establishing relationship between men, material, and machinery to carry on business efficiently for earning profits. This may be called the process of organising. The arrangement which follows this process of organising is called a business undertaking or organisation. A business undertaking can be better understood by analysing its characteristics. Business can be defined as an organization that provides goods and services to others who want or need them.

CHARACTERISTICS OF AN IDEAL FORM OF ORGANIZATION

The characteristics of an ideal form of organization are found in varying degrees in different forms of organization. The entrepreneur, while selecting a form of organization for his business, should consider the following factors.

1. Ease of formation: It should be easy to form the organization. The formation should not involve many legal formalities and it should not be time consuming.

2. Adequacy of Capital: The form of organization should facilitate the raising of the required amount of capital at a reasonable cost. If the enterprise requires a large amount of capital, the preconditions for attracting capital from the public are a) safety of investment b) fair return on investment and c) transferability of the holding.

3. Limit of Liability: A business enterprise may be organized on the basis of either limited or unlimited liability. From the point of view of risk, limited liability is preferable. It means that the liability of the owner as regards the debts of the business is limited only to the amount of capital agreed to be contributed by him. Unlimited liability means that even the owners' personal assets will be liable to be attached for the payment of the business debts.

4. Direct relationship between Ownership, Control and Management: The responsibility for management must be in the hands of the owners of the firm. If the owners have no control on the management, the firm may not be managed efficiently.

5. Continuity and Stability: Stability is essential for any business concern. Uninterrupted existence enables the entrepreneur to formulate long-term plans for the development of the business concern.

6. Flexibility of Operations: another ideal characteristic of a good form of organization is flexibility of operations. Changes may take place either in market conditions or the states' policy toward industry or in the conditions of supply of various factors of production. The nature of organization should be such as to be able to adjust itself to the changes without much difficulty.

1.3 FORMS OF BUSINESS ORGANIZATIONS

Sole Proprietorships. A sole proprietorship is the easiest organization to form or to understand. Most small businesses are or were originally sole proprietorships. Essentially, any business not of any other form is a proprietorship. It is the form of business started out by anyone who just starts a business. Proprietorships may be businesses as small as a child's lemonade stand or as large as a multi-billion dollar family held business.

Accounting for proprietorships is very simple. In practice, many small proprietorships even mix their owner's and the company's finances, but this is not ideal. The US government has created an income tax form "schedule C" to keep income separate, but it is still filed as part of the owner's individual's return; no separate business entity return needs to be filed.

Proprietorships often lack the sophistication of strategic planning, but that does not mean that they should not have it. Mission statements, strategic objectives and action plans are all key items that would benefit a small business as well as a large one, and may in fact be more important. Most small businesses fail – a fact that could change with better strategy. The strategy of many small businesses is either to make money (no strategy – just a fuzzy goal) or to keep the owner busy at something he or she likes (also not a strategy).

Advantages

a) Sole decision maker
b) Keep all the profits
c) Easy to start

Disadvantages

a) Limited money (capital) to start investment
b) No specialization which means a lot of work for owner
c) Severe financial risk with unlimited liability
d) Hard to attract workers looking for permanent work because long term future unsure

Appropriate for small market where good / service is not mass produced (e.g. accounting, dentistry, engineering)

Partnerships. These, at the base, are proprietorships whose ownerships are shared between two or more people. The other factors are the same, although many apparent partnerships can be actually small corporations that have a limited number of owners. Partnerships have advantages over proprietorships. Multiple owners mean that if one is not present (or ill), management may still continue in the business. If the right mix of owners exists, they can complement each other's skills. For example, one partner may be good at operations, another good at marketing, and another good at finance and so fourth. Putting multiple owners together can result in better decisions, as well. There are numerous examples of "two heads are better than one."

But partnerships can have drawbacks. This is too frequently the case when the partners do not get along. Personal goals and strategies may not be compatible. Anyone considering forming a partnership should at the same time consider how it would be dissolved. A common way is to include a "shotgun" clause in the documents that form the partnership. Basically, a shotgun clause is a pre-established way for one partner to buy out another. It is easiest set up with two partners, but any number can be involved. Insuring legality is critical. Any good business should have a solid relationship with an attorney who will prepare proper documents. Developing a method of ending a partnership before it forms should be part of the strategy of every would-be partner.

Advantages
a)   More capital can be raised
b)   Workload shared allowing for vacations and specialization
c)   Sounder business decisions can be made

Disadvantages
a)   Partners can have disagreements
b)   Unlimited liability for debt can hurt partner who is not responsible for poor business decisions
c)   When one partner dies or leaves a new partnership agreement must be made

Commonly found in farming, the professions (e.g. law), restaurants, construction and repair work

Unlimited life and limited liability

Proprietorships and partnerships are simple and easy to establish, but may not be the ideal form of an organization. Many people want their organizations to live on after they are through working in them. They may want to sell the ongoing business; they may hire professional management and take owner's profits without working in the organization; or they may use the business to employ family or friends, passing it down to younger generations.

Normally, proprietorships are part of their owner's lives. When their owners are though with them or die, proprietorships die, too. The organizations we just described with expectations for existing beyond their owner's lives should have lives of their own. There are several forms of organizations that gain legal lives of their own – limited partnerships; limited liability companies or partnerships; "C" corporations. All exist independently of their owners and can live on after the owners are through with them.

Limited Liability Company (LLC) or Limited Liability Partnership (LLP).

In the simplest form, these are essentially proprietorships with few partners, designed to obtain the liability limit of separating personal assets from the business. LLPs are frequently used by legal and medical practices, so that partners (owner-operators) may come and go, giving the organization life after the founders leave as well as protecting the owners from excessive liability.

Note that there is also a business form called a **limited partnership**. These are frequently established for investments. Oil and gas exploration and production, equipment leasing and other business entities are often established as investments. Limited partnership paperwork is much easier than setting up a corporation, liability is limited (for limited partners), and the investment may be for a limited time, such as the life of the equipment or oil well. There will be a general partner, however, who has a different liability. But even in this case, the general partner's liability may be limited by the form of business the general partner has taken.

Corporations:

This is the form of corporation with which we are most familiar. General Motors, Ford, Boeing, and most other big names are "C corps". C corporations allow an unlimited number of shareholders (owners), none of whom risk more than their investment in the stock of the organization. Typically, corporations intend to be around forever and have a most important goal of increasing the wealth of the people who own their stock. The negative of "C" corps is double taxation. The corporation pays taxes on profits it earns, then the shareholder pays taxes on either dividends paid by the corporation from its profits, or on the capital gains the shareholder receives upon selling the stock of a corporation that has been successful.

Advantages

a) Limited liability which means only personally liable for the amount of money you have invested in the company

b) Easier to raise capital for the business (e.g. retained earnings, securities like preferred & common shares, bonds)

c) Longevity

d) Specialization through mass production

Disadvantages

a) Unaccountable management may act selfishly against the best interests of the shareholders

b) Management less motivated to be successful if they don't have ownership stake in company

c) Expensive to establish

d) Double taxation

Stock Market is an organized market where corporations can sell shares or ownership in their company

OTHER FORMS OF BUSINESS ORGANIZATIONS

There are other forms of businesses or combinations of businesses. Many of these are actually combinations of businesses that allow one business to significantly influence another. Listed below are the most common:

License: A license is a right given by one organization to use some of its assets (usually intellectual - like brand names, technology, etc.) to another organization. For example, one firm may make a product that is under patent or uses a hard-to-copy technology from another. The licensee the company that does not have the technology but would like to pay a "royalty," typically a percentage of sales, to the original property owner or licensor. The licensee and the licensor are independent companies and may be corporations or other forms of business themselves. The terms of the license will give the licensor rights over how the licensee does business, even though the licensee is a separate business. This is done to protect the licensor.

Franchise: This is a special license from one organization to another to operate the business in great measure determined by the granting organization. For example, a licensee may own a motel that operates as a Holliday Inn. The motel owner has bought a franchise and will pay a fee to Holliday Inn. The ownership form of the motel could also be a proprietorship, partnership or a corporation as can be the franchise grantor. Note that when the franchise agreement ends, the owner still has a motel, just that it will not be part of the Holliday Inn family from that time on (depending on the franchise agreement).

Joint Venture: This is a business combination of two or more companies that creates a third company to perform a specific function or to handle a specific business. Ownership of the joint venture belongs to both (or all) parent companies. The joint venture is a new company formed from assets, including employees, from the parent companies. Employees in the joint venture are typically new employees for the joint venture. For example, different and new employee retirement plans may exist. Frequently the employees are given their seniority from their old organizations for vacation or other non-retirement purposes.

Joint Stock Company: A company which has some features of a corporation and some features of a partnership. The company sells fully transferable stock, but all shareholders have unlimited liability.

The main advantages of Joint Stock Company are –

    a. Large financial resources

    b. Limited Liability:

    c. Professional management:

    d. Large-scale production

    e. Contribution to society:

    f. Research and Development

Limitations of Joint Stock Company

    a. Difficult to form:

    b. Excessive government control

    c. Delay in policy decisions

    d. Concentration of economic power and wealth in few hands

Strategic Alliance: In this case, two or more organizations agree to work together to accomplish a goal. For example, one company may manufacture a product but have poor marketing, so it forms a strategic alliance with a marketing company. The terms, which organization gets what amount of profit, etc., will be negotiated, but neither gives up any ownership to the other or a third party.

There are other forms of business relationships, but these cover the most common and should provide a background for studying strategy. Note that the terms "corporation," "organization," "firm" and "company" are used almost interchangeably. The strategic considerations we make here apply to all, even non-profit organizations.

Selecting the form of your business depends on several factors. The logic is:

1. Select a form that limits liability.

2. Consider the long range implications of the forms that you are considering, especially tax implications.

3. Discuss the pros and cons and the costs of set-up with your attorney and tax advisor/ accountant. Together select the best form for you.

4. Complete the appropriate paperwork. Total cost should be under $1,000.

> Note that a business can begin as a sole proprietorship or partnership an then change forms to one with limited liability later. This is an acceptabl strategy providing that there is little liability exposure during the initial period. Liability insurance will need to be acquired in any case, as the insurance company lawyers will deal with potential liability claims if they arise, leaving you more time to manage your business no matter how your company is formed. But insurance does not take the place of the limited

1.4   CHARACTERISTIC   FEATURES   OF   BUSINESS ORGANIZATIONS

CHARACTE-RISTICS	PROPRIETOR-SHIPS	GENERAL PARTNERSHIP	LIMITED PARTNERSHIP	CORPORATIONS, CLOSED AND GENERAL
Method of creation	Start your business	Created by agreement of the parties	Same and file statutory form in public	Charter issued by state
Liability of members	Owner has limited personal liability	Partners have unlimited liability	General partners — unlimited liability; Limited partners — limited liability	Shareholders have limited liability
Duration	Termination by death, bankruptcy,	Termination by death, agreement, bankruptcy or withdrawal of a partner	The term provided in the certificate	May be perpetual

CHARACTERI-STICS	PROPRIETOR-SHIPS	GENERAL PARTNERSHIP	LIMITED PARTNERSHIP	CORPORATIONS, CLOSED AND GENERAL
Transferability of interest	Generally by sale of assets	Not transferable except by agreement of all partners	General Partner - not transferable, limited partner – transferable	Generally freely transferable subject to limited contacts between shareholders
Management	Owner has absolute control	All partners, in absence of agreement have equal voice	General Partner — equal voice Limited partners - very limited voice	Shareholders elect directors who set policy
Taxation	Not a taxable entity; net income taxed to owner	Not a taxable entity; net income taxed to partners whether distributed or not	Same	Income taxed to corporations; dividends taxed to shareholders
Legal entity for progress of: a) suit in firm name b) owning property in firm name c) bankruptcy d) limited liability	By modern law is an entity for: a) yes b) yes c) Yes d) No	By modern law is an entity for: a) yes b) yes c) Yes d) No	Same d) General partners - no, limited -yes	Is a legal entity in all states for all purposes
Transact business in other states	No limitation	No limitation	Copy of certificate must be filed in all counties where doing business	Must qualify to do business and obtain certificate of authority
Organization fee, annual license fee and annual reports.	None	None	Minimum franchise tax per year	All required
Modification of amendment of articles	No requirement	No requirement	Must file changes	Must obtain state approval
Agency Owners / operators	None Are not employees	Each partner is both principal and agent of his co-partners Partners are not employees	General partners - same as in general partners; limited partners - not principals or agents	A shareholder is not an agent of the corporation Officers are employees

1.5 PUBLIC SECTOR ENTERPRISES AND TYPES

A **government-owned corporation, state-owned enterprise** or **government business enterprise** is a legal entity created by a government to undertake commercial or business activities on behalf of an owner government. There is no standard definition of a government-owned corporation (GOC) or state-owned enterprise (SOE), although the two terms can be used inter-changeably.

The term **government-linked company** (GLC) is sometimes used to refer to corporate entities that may be private or public (listed on a stock exchange) where an existing government owns a stake using a holding company. There are two main definitions of GLCs are dependent on the proportion of the corporate entity a government owns. One definition purports that a company is classified as a GLC if a government owns an effective controlling interest (>50%), while the second definition suggests that any corporate entity that has a government as a shareholder is a GLC.

A **quasi-governmental** *organization, corporation, business,* or *agency*) is an entity that is treated by national laws and regulations to be under the guidance of the government, but also separate and autonomous from the government. While the entity may receive some revenue from charging customers for its services, these organizations are often partially or majorly funded by the government. They are usually considered highly important to smooth running of society, and are sometimes propped up with cash infusions in times of crisis to help surmount situations that would bankrupt a normal privately-owned business. They may also possess law-enforcement authority, usually related to their functions.

List of Some Central PSUs(PUBLIC SECTOR UNITS)

- Bharat Electronics Limited (BEL)
- Rail India Technical and Economic Services (RITES)
- Hindustan Aeronautics Limited (HAL)
- Indian Oil Corporation Limited (IOCL)
- Oil and Natural Gas Corporation (ONGC)
- Bharat Heavy Electricals Limited (BHEL)
- National Thermal Power Corporation (NTPC)
- Power Finance Corporation Limited (PFC)
- Steel Authority of India Limited (SAIL)

- Bharat Sanchar Nigam Limited (BSNL)
- Bharat Petroleum Corporation Limited (BPCL)
- Hindustan Petroleum Corporation Limited (HPCL)
- Gas Authority of India Limited (GAIL)
- Mangalore Refineries and Petrochemicals Limited (MRPL)

HINDUSTAN ANTIBIOTICS LIMITED (HAL)

HAL is the first public sector undertaking in the Drugs & Pharmaceutical Sector. HAL was setup in cooperation with the WHO and UNICEF with the social objective of providing affordable drugs through out India. The plant was commissioned in 1955-56. The undertaking with its plant at Pimpri, Pune is engaged in the manufacture of bulk drugs, mainly Penicillins, Streptomycin and a number of formulations. HAL has also four joint sector undertakings of which three units have been promoted in collaboration with the respective State Governments and one with a private sector company. These are:

1. Maharashtra Antibiotics & Pharmaceuticals Limited   (MAPL)
2. Karnataka Antibiotics & Pharmaceuticals Limited   (KAPL)
3. Manipur State Drugs & Pharmaceuticals Limited   (MSDPL)
4. Hindustan MAX-GB, Pimpri,Pune   (HM-GB)

INDIAN DRUGS AND PHARMACEUTICALS LIMITED

IDPL is the largest Central Pharma Public Sector Undertaking in India with plants at Rishikesh, Gurgaon, Chennai, Hyderabad and Muzaffarpur. The IDPL was incorporated in 1961 with main objectives of creating self-sufficiency in respect of essential life saving medicines, to free the country from dependence on imports and to provide medicines to the millions at affordable prices and not to make millions from the medicines. IDPL was basically conceived and established as a part of Healthcare Infrastructure and has played a pioneering infra-structural role in the growth of Indian Drug Industry base.

IDPL played a major role in the strategic National Health Programmes like Family Welfare Programme & Population Control (Mala-D & Mala-N) anti-malarials (Chloroquine) and prevention of dehydration (ORS) by providing quality medicines. During the country's calamity of outbreak of Plague in 1994, IDPL was the only company which played the sheet anchor role in supplying Tetracycline for the entire Nation. Similarly, company had made uninterrupted supply of Chloroquine to combat.

1.6 CHANGING BUSINESS ENVIRONMENT IN POST-LIBERALIZATION SCENARIO.

The economic boom that is being experienced in India is largely attributed to the globalization and liberalization of the Indian economy. The era prior to the 1990s was quite averse to the concept of an open market policy and the Indian markets were predominantly closed in nature. The government of India, however, ruled and regulated Indian markets but with the globalization and liberalization of the Indian economy, the whole market scenario changed in no time. The economic policy drafted in early 1990s by the government of India facilitated huge inflow of Foreign Direct Investment (FDI) and Foreign Institutional Investors (FII) in to the much insulated Indian markets. Prime economic factors like Industrial Growth, Balance-of-Payments, Merchandise Exports, Invisible Accounts and Foreign-Exchange-Reserves witnessed positive growth and effected tremendous growth of Indian Economy.

The positive effects of globalization and liberalization of Indian economy can be corroborated from the following facts -

- **Industrial Growth** - for the first time has exceeded 10%. Manufacturing growth rate has exceeded 12% in 6 months (April-September, 2006). The mining and quarrying sector has registered a growth of 4%. The electricity sector recorded a double-digit growth of 12% during September, 2006 as compared to September, 2005. Consumer durables and non-durables have also recorded upswings. The use-base economic sub-groups and intermediate goods have registered an impressive growth of almost 15% during September, 2006 over September, 2005. Consumer goods have recorded a high growth of 13%. The National Manufacturing Competitiveness Council has targeted 12 to 14% growth in the 11th Plan period.

- **Foreign Institutional Investors (FIIs)** - net investments in equities crossed US$ 7 billion in calendar 2006. FII net investment till 6 November 2006 has been US$ 7.08 billion. according to the Securities and Exchange Board of India. 151 new FIIs have opened their offices in India during first 10 months of 2006. The total number of FIIs in India stands at 974 as on November, 2006 Foreign Direct Investment (FDI) - India envisage of attracting $10 billion of foreign direct investment (FDI) this year as inflows have nearly doubled to US$ 4.4 billion in April-September 2006. India has recorded its highest rise in salaries at 22% in the first half of 2006-07 against increase of 17% in 2005-06

- India's economy grew at 9.3% in quarter April-June and it was driven by manufacturing, construction and services sector and agriculture sector

- GDP factor for the first quarter of 2007-08 was at Rs 7,23,132 crore, registering a growth rate of 9.3% over the corresponding quarter of previous year

- Manufacturing industry registered 11.9% growth

- Electricity, gas, and water supply performed well and recorded an impressive growth rate of 8.3%

- Trade, hotels, transport and communication registered a growth rate of 12%

- Financing, insurance, real estate and business services recorded an impressive growth rate of at 11% during the 1st quarter of this fiscal

- The growth rate of agriculture, forestry & fishing' and 'mining & quarrying' are estimated at 3.8 per cent, and 3.2 per cent, respectively during the 1st quarter of 2007-2008

- Exports grew by 18.11% during the 1st quarter of 2007-2008 and the imports shoot up by 34.30% during the same period

- India's FOREX reserves (excluding Gold and SDRs) stood at $219.75 billion at the end of July ' 07

- Merchandise Exports recorded strong growth

These upswings of indicators are the result of globalization and liberalization of Indian economy introduced and implemented in the early 1990s. With consistent rise of the manufacturing and service sector activities together with bullish stock market the growth story of the Indian economy is expected to rise further and help India achieve its economic goals.

The rapid **scientific technological advancements** are reshaping the world. Developments in information and communication technology have revolutionized every activity, be it scientific or business and commerce or individual and personal.

In the opinion of some experts the twenty first century competition is characterized by at least three fundamental paradigms shifts, viz. -

(a) Ability of organisations and individuals to network globally and seamlessly;

(b) Ability to communicate, transmit, store and retrieve large amounts to information including voice, data, video; and

(c) Mobility of capital to feed good projects around the world.

With the battle for market share and mind-share deepening, companies are increasingly resorting to non-traditional resources (like knowledge) and innovative means (like quick response) to create sustainable competitive advantage.

DEVELOPMENTS IN BUSINESS SCENARIO

a. The New Economic Policy (NEP) of 1991, announced by the Government of India. This is a landmark year in the sphere of economic liberalization and trade related reforms. A number of innovative changes have taken place in the business environment. Major areas of reforms related to abolition of industrial licensing system except for a short list, opening up of Indian economy to foreign investment, liberlisation of norms for foreign technology transfer, abolition of Chapter III of the MRTP Act relating to concentration of economic power, intention of the Government to adopt a new approach to Public Sector Undertakings including disinvestments etc. With these policy re-orientation, the role of the Government, as the regulator has changed from exercising control to one of providing help and guidance by making essential procedures fully transparent and eliminating delays.

b. Simplification and raitonalisation of both direct and indirect tax laws including lowering of tariff barriers and removal of quantitative restrictions.Abolition of the office of the Controller of Capital Issues and the setting up of Securities and Exchange Board of India (SEBI), as an autonomous body to promote, regulate and develop the capital market on healthy lines and protection of investor's interests in securities. A number of Rules and Regulations have been issued by SEBI for regulating the activities of intermediaries/others in the capital market.

c. Replacement of Foreign Exchange Regulations Act, 1973 by Foreign Exchange Management Act, 2000 including introduction of convertibility of rupees on current account.

d. Liberalization of norms for Foreign Direct Investment (FDI) in Indian Industries and also portfolio investment norms.

e. Issue of regulations by SEBI regarding SEBI (Prohibition of Insider Trading) Regulations, 1992, SEBI (Prohibition of Fraudulent and Unfair Practices relating to Securities Market) Regulations, 1995 and SEBI (Substantial Acquisition of Shares and Takeovers) Regulations, 1997 as amended from time to time.

f. Setting up of World Trade Organisation (WTO) as an apex body at the international level, to which India is a signatory, to regulate and develop international trade on healthy lines.

g. Replacement of MRTP Act, 1969 by Competition Act of 2002.

Globalisation of Indian economy and substantial reduction of tariff barriers-these are pointers to the changing business environment. These factors have given rise to increasing competition in the market place for the Indian products and services. There is an imperative need to manufacture and market high quality products which can withstand the products of foreign manufacturers. The fast changing business environment calls for a new approach to the management of corporate organisations.

SUMMARY:

In this unit, meaning of business and organisation are discussed followed by characteristic features of business. The various types of business organisation are Sole proprietorship, partnership, joint stock company and public enterprises. Finally post liberalisation business environment is discussed.

REVIEW QUESTIONS:

1. What do you mean by Business or Organisation?
2. Explain the various functions of business organizations with examples
3. What are the basic characteristics of ideal forms of organizations?
4. What are the different forms organizations? Explain in detail
5. Distinguish between the sole proprietary and partnership concerns
6. Compare and contrast the joint stock companies and public enterprises in India
7. Highlight the post-liberalized economic progress in India
8. Discuss the different opportunities and challenges are in front of business organizations
9. What are the advantages and disadvantages of sole proprietary, partnership, cooperative and Public organizations.

Chapter 2

MANUFACTURING MANAGEMENT

2.1 INTRODUCTION

Manufacturing is the use of machines, tools and labor to make things for use or sale. The term may refer to a range of human activity, from handicraft to high tech, but is most commonly applied to industrial production, in which raw materials are transformed into finished goods on a large scale. Such finished goods may be used for manufacturing other, more complex products, such as household appliances or automobiles, or sold to wholesalers, who in turn sell them to retailers, who then sell them to end users - the "consumers".

Manufacturing Management involves the philosophies, strategies, tactics, methods and techniques that enable managers of manufacturing to achieve low unit cost, superb quality, great flexibility and innovation. This field builds on the concept of quality and the philosophy of striving continually to achieve the highest possible organization-wide standards.

Modern manufacturing includes all intermediate processes required for the production and integration of a product's components. Some industries, such as semiconductor and steel manufacturers use the term **fabrication** instead.

The manufacturing sector is closely connected with engineering and industrial design. Examples of major manufacturers in the United States include General Motors Corporation, Ford Motor Company, Chrysler, Boeing, Gates Rubber Company and Pfizer. Examples in Europe include Airbus, Daimler, BMW, Fiat, and Michelin Tyre.

Lean Manufacturing

The term "lean" was coined to describe Toyota's business during the late 1980s by a research team headed by Jim Womack, Ph.D., at MIT's International Motor Vehicle Program. "Lean manufacturing is the system which aims in elimination of the waste from the system with a systematic and continuous approach".

Companies are always searching for a more efficient way to run their business. Cutting cost is one of the more popular ways of getting ahead of the competition. This is the proper management setting where the principles of lean manufacturing can be put to good use.

Lean manufacturing is the management philosophy of no waste. This method focuses upon reducing waste in a manufacturing business or any other type of business. The seven wastes are over-production, over-processing, transportation, motion, inventory, waiting time and defects. These lean manufacturing principles serve as a guide for any company that wants to have peak performance in their organization. These principles can create a more productive work environment, no matter if it is in a warehouse, factory or the office.

2.2 MANUFACTURING AND PRODUCTION MANAGEMENT

Earlier production management was considered as manufacturing management but today manufacturing and service organisations come under the category of production management, broadly known as operation management

In production, the raw material is not procured from outside, the company owns it and after processing and make the final product. But in Manufacturing, the company procures the raw material from outside, and then makes the final product. Manufacturing is the art of streamlining production.

Manufacturing is a process of converting raw material in to finished product by using various processes, machines and energy. It is a narrow term. Production is a process of converting inputs in to outputs. Every type of manufacturing is production but every production is not a manufacturing. For example, making of a turbine by various processes is manufacturing, assemble the various parts to make a engine is production not manufacturing. Manufacturing includes other stages such as design, sales, management and marketing.

Production Management

"Production" involves the step-by-step conversion of one form of materials into another through chemical or mechanical processing to create or enhance the utility of the products or services.

The word 'production management' arrived first with the emergence of manufacturing industry and the necessity to manage it as such. The meaning of the term "production management" is clarified in the following definitions:

(1) According to MJ.S. Harry, *the word production is often used to mean the same as manufacture. In order to go through a process of manufacturing itself, we need basically three things: someone to do the job, his equipment and the necessary materials. To run production, we require service activities which make sure that the manufacturing activity can go on and control to make sure that it goes in the right direction.*

(2) According to E.S. Buffa, "*Production management deals with decision-making related to production processes so that the resulting goods or service is produced according to specifications, in the amounts and by the schedule demanded and at minimum cost.*"

The definition given by E.S.Buffa is simple, clear and exhaustive. It explains the following important aspects of production management.

(a)   It is a decision-making managerial function;

(b)   The decisions are made regarding the production processes required for converting the raw materials into finished products, and

(c)   The production or output should be according to specifications, in the specified quantities, as per the schedule and at minimum cost.

A production system takes inputs and converts them into outputs. The conversion process is the predominant activity of a production system. The primary concern of an operations manager is the activities of the conversion process. Operations Management concerns itself with the conversion of inputs into outputs, using physical resources, so as to provide the desired utility (utilities) of form, place, possession or state or a combination thereof – to the customer while meeting the other organizational objectives of effectiveness, efficiency and adaptability. It distinguishes itself from the other functions such as personnel, marketing etc. by its primary concern for "conversion by using physical resources."

Production and Operations

These days therefore both manufacturing and service organizations fall into the scope of production management. Thus production management which was formerly considered as manufacturing management only, now after inclusion of services into its scope, is broadly known as operations management. Many non-manufacturing organizations providing services like hospitals, banks, transportation, farming, warehousing etc. are now covered by operations management.

Operations in the services organizations have some unique features, different from those which has manufacturing base. These are:

(1)   Non-inventorial output of service, since generally no stock is produced.

(2)   Variable demand.

(3)   Labour-intensive operations mostly.

(4)   Location of service is dictated by the location of the users.

Operations managers are responsible for producing the supply of goods or services in organizations. Operations managers make decisions regarding the operations function and the transformation systems used. Operations management is the study of decision making in the operations function.

GOALS OF PRODUCTION MANAGEMENT

Production involves the things which are essential for the manufacture of products. The objective of Production Management is to produce the desired product or specified product by specified methods so that the optimal utilization of available resources is met with. Hence the production management is responsible to produce the desired product, which has marketability at the cheapest price by proper planning, the manpower, material and processes. Production management must see that it will deliver right goods of right quantity at right place and at right price. When the above objective is achieved, we say that we have effective Production Management system.

The Goals/ Objectives of the production management are 'to produce goods services of right quality and quantity at the right time and right manufacturing cost'.

1. Right quality

The quality of product is established based upon the customers needs. The right quality is not necessarily best quality. It is determined by the cost of the product and the technical characteristics as suited to the specific requirements.

2. Right quantity

The manufacturing organization should produce the products in right number. If they are produced in excess of demand the capital will block up in the form of inventory and if the quantity is produced in short of demand, leads to shortage of products.

3. Right time

Timeliness of delivery is one of the important parameter to judge the effectiveness of production department. So, the production department has to make the optimal utilization of input resources to achieve its objective.

4. Right manufacturing cost

Manufacturing costs are established before the product is actually manufactured. Hence, all attempts should be made to produce the products at pre-established cost, so as to reduce the variation between actual and the standard (pre-established) cost.

2.3 ELEMENTS OF PRODUCTION & OPERATION

Managing operations can be enclosed in a frame of general management.Operation managers are concerned with planning, organizing, and controlling the activities which affect human behavior through models.

1. Planning

Activities that establishes a course of action and guide future decision-making is planning. The operations manager defines the objectives for the operations subsystem of the organization, and the policies, and procedures for achieving the objectives. This stage includes clarifying the role and focus of operations in the organization's overall strategy. It also involves product planning, facility designing and using the conversion process.

2. Organizing

Activities that establishes a structure of tasks and authority. Operation managers establish a structure of roles and the flow of information within the operations subsystem. They determine the activities required to achieve the goals and assign authority and responsibility for carrying them out.

3. Controlling

Activities that assure the actual performance in accordance with planned performance. To ensure that the plans for the operations subsystems are accomplished, the operations manager must exercise control by measuring actual outputs and comparing them to planned operations management. Controlling costs, quality, and schedules are the important functions here.

4. Behaviour

Operation managers are concerned with how their efforts to plan, organize, and control affect human behavior. They also want to know how the behavior of subordinates can affect management's planning, organizing, and controlling actions. Their interest lies in decision-making behavior.

5. Models

As operation managers plan, organize, and control the conversion process, they encounter many problems and must make many decisions. They can simplify their difficulties using models like aggregate planning models for examining how best to use existing capacity in short-term, break even analysis to identify break even volumes, linear programming and computer simulation for capacity utilization, decision tree analysis for long-term capacity problem of facility expansion, simple median model for determining best locations of facilities etc.

2.4 PRODUCTION PLANNING and CONTROL (PPC)

PPC comprise the planning, routing, dispatching in the manufacturing process so that the movement of material, performance of machines and operation of labour however are subdivided and are directed and coordinated as to quantity, quality, time and place. Planning and control are two basic and interrelated managerial functions

Preplanning, Planning & Control

The activities of preplanning, planning and control may be considered to take place in a time sequence. The preplanning is completed before production commences. Planning takes place immediately before production starts and control is exercised during production.

Preplanning:

It is the procedure followed in developing and designing a work or production of a developing and installing a proper layout or tools. It may be involved many functions of the organization and draws upon forecasting, product design, jigs and tool design, machine selection and estimating to enable proper design to be made. In short, preplanning decides what shall be made and how it shall be made. In respective manufacture a large uneconomic output could be produced if preplanning is omitted. It is also important in one of the operations such as setting up a new plants as preplanning can identify and avoid probable costly errors.

Planning:

This stage decides where and when the product shall be made. It includes the sequencing of operations viz. outing and the time schedule for manufacturing viz scheduling. It also states procedures for material planning and supplies, machine loading and deliveries. To perform as functions properly it will need past records of performance and to control statistic which may be obtained from pre-planning, cost control or progress.

Control:

This refers to the stage of ensuring that the planned action is in tact carried out. Control initiates the plan at the right time using dispatching and there after control makes appropriate adjustments through progressing to take care of any unforeseen circumstances

THE FUNCTIONS OF PPC

a. **Materials:** The selection of materials for the product. Production manager must have sound knowledge of materials and their properties, so that he can select appropriate materials for his product. Research on materials is necessary to find alternatives to satisfy the changing needs of the design in the product and availability of material resumes.

b. **Methods:** Finding the best method for the process, to search for the methods to suit the available resources, identifying the sequence of process are some of the activities of Production Management.

c.   **Machines and Equipment:** Selection of suitable machinery for the process desired, designing the maintenance policy and design of layout of machines are taken care of by the Production Management department.

d. **Estimating:** To fix up the Production targets and delivery dates and to keep the production costs at minimum, production management department does a thorough estimation of Production times and production costs. In competitive situation this will help the management to decide what should be done in arresting the costs at desired level.

e. **Loading and Scheduling:** The Production Management department has to draw the time table for various production activities, specifying when to start and when to finish the process required. It also has to draw the timings of materials movement and plan the activities of manpower. The scheduling is to be done keeping in mind the loads on hand and capacities of facilities available.

f.   Routing: This is the most important function of Production Management department. The Routing consists of fixing the flow lines for various raw materials, components etc., from the stores to the packing of finished product, so that all concerned knows what exactly is happening on the shop floor.

g.   Dispatching: The Production Management department has to prepare various documents such as Job Cards, Route sheets, Move Cards, Inspection Cards for each and every component of the product. These are prepared in a set of five copies. These documents are to be released from Production Management department to give green signal for starting the production. The activities of the shop floor will follow the instructions given in these documents. Activity of releasing the document is known as dispatching.

h.   Expediting or Follow up: Once the documents are dispatched, the management wants to know whether the activities are being carried out as per the plans or not. Expediting engineers go round the production floor along with the plans, compare the actual with the plan and feed back the progress of the work to the management. This will help the management to evaluate the plans.

i.   Inspection: Here inspection is generally concerned with the inspection activities during production, but a separate quality control department does the quality inspection, which is not under the control of Production Management. This is true because, if the quality inspection is given to production Management, then there is a chance of qualifying the defective products also. For example Teaching and examining of students is given to the same person, then there is a possibility of passing all the students in the first grade. To avoid this situation an external person does correction of answer scripts, so that the quality of answers are correctly judged.

j.   Evaluation: The Production department must evaluate itself and its contribution in fulfilling the corporate objectives and the departmental objectives. This is necessary for setting up the standards for future. What ever may be the size of the firm; Production management department alone must do Routing, Scheduling, Loading, dispatching and expediting. This is because this department knows very well regarding materials, Methods, and available resources etc. If the firms are small, all the above-mentioned functions are tono be carried out by Production Management Department. In medium sized firms in addition to Routing, Scheduling and Loading, Dispatching and expediting, some more functions like Methods, Machines may be under the control of Production Management Department. In large firms, there will be Separate departments for Methods, Machines, Materials and others but routing, loading and scheduling are the sole functions of Production Management.

All the above ten functions are categorized in three stage, that is Preplanning, Planning and control stages as shown in the following figures

PPC Phases

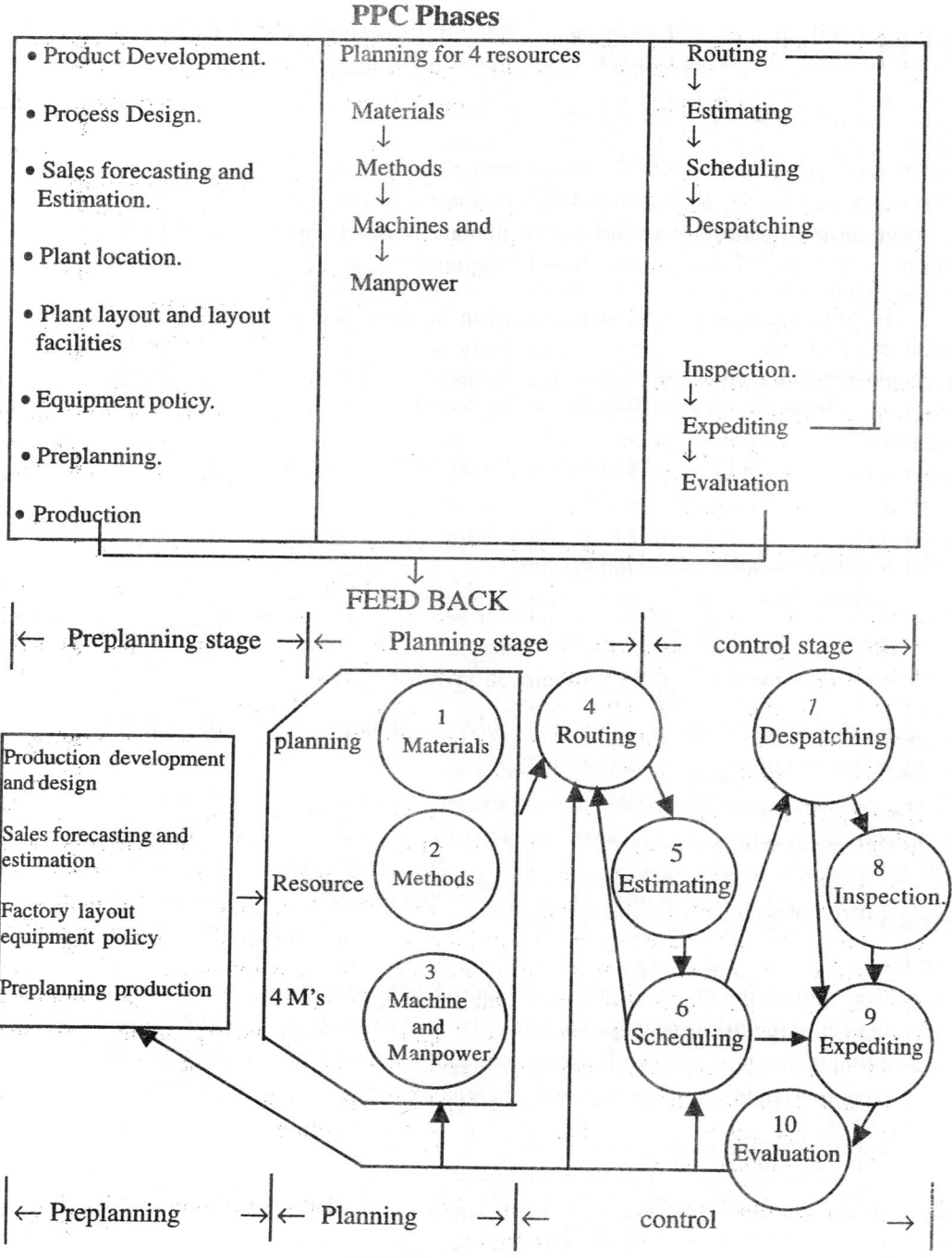

	Planning for 4 resources	Routing
• Product Development.		↓
• Process Design.	Materials	Estimating
	↓	↓
• Sales forecasting and Estimation.	Methods ↓	Scheduling ↓
	Machines and	Despatching
• Plant location.	↓	
	Manpower	
• Plant layout and layout facilities		
• Equipment policy.		Inspection. ↓
• Preplanning.		Expediting ↓
• Production		Evaluation

FEED BACK

← Preplanning stage → ← Planning stage → ← control stage →

PPC Function

2.5 PLANT LOCATION

Facility design involves determining the capacity, location, and layout for the facility. Capacity is a measure of an organization's ability to provide the demanded services or goods in the quantity requested by the customer and in a timely manner. Capacity planning involves estimating demand, determining the capacity of facilities, and deciding how to change the organization's capacity to respond to demand. Facility location is the placement of a facility with respect to its customers and suppliers.

Facility location is a strategic decision because it is a long term commitment of resources that cannot easily or inexpensively be changed. When evaluating a location, management should consider: customer convenience, initial investment for land and facilities, government incentives, operating costs, and transportation costs. In addition, qualitative factors, such as recreational activities for employees, adequate transportation infrastructure, and a favorable labor environment may be important. Facility layout is the arrangement of the work space within a facility. It considers which departments or work areas should be adjacent to one another so that the flow of product, information, and people can move quickly and efficiently through the production system.

Plant location decisions are very important because they have direct bearing on factors like, financial, employment and distribution patterns. In the long run, relocation of plant may even benefit the organization. But, the relocation of the plant involves stoppage of production, and also cost for shifting the facilities to a new location. In addition to these things, it will introduce some inconvenience in the normal functioning of the business. Hence, at the time of starting any industry, one should generate several alternate sites for locating the plant. After a critical analysis, the best site is to be selected for commissioning the plant. Location of warehouses and other facilities are also having direct bearing on the operational performance of organizations.

Reasons for plant location study.

The following events are quite common in any business venture.
- Establishment of a new venture.
- Expansion of existing business.
- Significant change in existing demand, supply and marketing locations.
- Significant change in the cost structure.
- Government policies

Because of these events, an organization will be keen in additional or alternate sites for its production activities. So, the plant location becomes an important decision which in turn influences plant layout and facilities needed. Also, it influences capital investment and operating costs. For example, in steel industry, if we integrate the units' right from ore extraction to final steel formation in a nearby area, the transportation cost would be substantially reduced and also, the reliability of supplies to the final stages of production in the integrated plant would be improved. This in turn, improves the productivity of the plant.

Facilities planning

Facilities planning have four main components: geographic location, structure and specific site, equipment choice, and layout.

Facilities are the plant and the office within which Operations Management does its work. In addition to the buildings and the spaces that are built, bought, or rented, facilities also include equipment used in the plant and the office. There are four main components of facilities planning and they strongly interact with each other. These four are

1. **Location of facilities**. Where, in the geographic sense, should the various operations be located? Where is it best to..." fabricated assemble each product, locate the service center, situate the sales offices, and position the administration?

    Many location factors have to be dealt with in a qualitative fashion. Common sense prevails. Qualitative factors such as being near supplies of raw materials and/or sources of skilled labor vie with being close to customers. Seldom can all desires be satisfied. The options may be to choose one over the other or to compromise with an in-between location. There are similar problems for distributors who want to be located close by all kinds of transportation facilities (road, rail, airports, and marine docks).

    Other location factors are better dealt with in a quantitative fashion because common sense does not work. The reason is that some real problems are too big to grasp all of the possible options. Because of this, optimal location assignments are often counterintuitive. For example, if a transportation analysis is made manageable by dividing the problem into regional sub-problems, the solution may be seriously sub-optimal (far from being the best that is possible). The systems approach, which endeavors to include all relevant factors, is needed in this case.

2. **Structure and specific site selection:** In what kind of facility should the process be located? How should the building or space be chosen? Is it best for the company to build the facility, buy, or rent it? Choice of a specific building is often decided after the location is chosen. However, there are circumstances where the location, site, and structure should be considered together. This makes structure and site decisions complex problems best resolved by using the systems approach.

3. **Equipment choice**. What kind of process technology is to be used? This decision often dominates structure and site options. In turn, there may be environmental factors that limit the choice of locations. Equipment choice can include transport systems and available routes. Interesting systems problems arise that combine all three aspects of facilities planning.

4. **Layout of the facility**. Where should machines and people be placed in the plant or office? There is interaction of equipment choice with layout, structure, site, and location. The size of the facility is determined by both current needs and future projections to allow for growth. Thus, facilities planning are systems planning. Once the location, site, and structure are determined, layout details can be decided.

Factors affecting location

One of the important problems of launching an industrial enterprise is the choice of suitable location which will help in minimization of production cost and maximization of profit. In order to select an optimum location, the promoters must carefully study the impact of the following factors.

(i) Availability of Raw Materials : The availability of the required quantity of raw materials at a reasonable cost is an important factor for determining the location of an industrial unit. In most of the industries, the cost of raw materials forms more than 50% of the total cost of their products. The impact of raw materials on location depends upon their nature and the source of their deposits. Weber classified raw materials into ubiquities and localized materials. Generally, ubiquities like water, clay, and sand which are found at all places have very little influence on location. That means the place of production would be fixed independently. But in some cases materials of ubiquitous nature may so vary in quantity and quality that are in fact regarded as fixed. For example, paper manufacturing plants require a regular supply of a large quantity of pure water and they are, therefore, located neat the banks of rivers. Localized raw materials may be further sub-divided into pure materials such as raw cotton and wool and gross materials such as sugarcane, iron ore and coal. The latter type of materials lose their weight in the process of production. If a large quantity of weight losing material is to be used during production, it is better to locate the plant near the source of material because there will be greater savings of transportation costs. For instance, iron and steel industry, which uses coal and iron ore as raw materials has localized near the coal and iron ore mines.

(ii) Labour Supply : Every plant requires an adequate supply of labour with appropriate skills. Weber deduced that an industrial unit will deviate form the point of minimum transportation cost to the cheaper labour centre if the additional cost of transportation at the new centre is more than compensated by the savings in labour cost. But this hypothesis has lost its significance in the recent years because of many reasons. Labour is easily mobile and there is a level of minimum wages fixed by law below which an industrial concern cannot go. Moreover, certain industries are capital intensive and they require less labour. Therefore, it can be said that supply of labour, particularly in a country where there is large scale unemployment, is not as important as it used to be half a century ago.

(iii) Proximity to the Market : Industrial units using non-weight losing raw materials tend to locate near the market because of so many advantages. A manufacture can improve his customer relations and render rapid services to his customers. Industries producing perishable commodities and those producing for a local market are also drawn towards the market, because it would reduce the cost of transport in distributing the finished products. The industrial units tend to disperse only if they find a new market for their products.

(iv) Transport Facilities : Transport service are required for assembling of material and distribution of products. While selecting the location it should be seen that transportation facilities are easily available at reasonable rates. The junction points of waterways, roadways and railways have the tendency to become industrial centers because of this reason only. If an industrial unit is directly linked with the means of transportation, its transportation costs are lower. Besides transportation, communication service also plays an important role in the location of industrial units. Every business firm requires information as regards raw materials, finished goods and market price which can be made available only when there are communication facilities. Since transport and communication facilities are not adequately available in rural areas, entrepreneurs are reluctant to start their operations in those areas.

(v) Power and Fuel : An Adequate supply of power and fuel is an important factor for the un-interrupted operations of any enterprise. In the initial days of industrial revolution, industrial units were located near coal deposits because coal was the major source of power and fuel and was of weight losing nature and quite bulky. But with the introduction of other sources of power like electricity, gas, oil, etc., the power factor has become more mobile. This has helped in dispersal of industries. The industrial units which mainly depend on electric power tend to shift from a place if they do not get its regular supply. But iron and steel industry where coal is still the major source of fuel is located near the coal mines.

(vi) Climatic Considerations : Natural and climatic considerations like level of ground, topography (hilly and rocky surface) of a region, and drainage facilities influence the location of industries in certain cases. For example, cotton textile mills require a humid climate. The humid climate of Bombay offered greater scope for the development of cotton textile in dustry. But the development of artificial humidification and air-conditioning has reduced the importance of climate to same extent. Enterpreneurs do not prefer to locate their units in hilly and rocky areas because of increase in transport cost. Similarly, regions which are subject to frequent floods, earth-quakes, etc., do not attract industrial units.

(vii) Supply of Capital : Finance is the life-blood of any industrial venture. Availability of adequate funds at low rates of interests is an important factor influencing industrial location. But in these days capital has become a highly mobile factor of production. Despite this fact, availability of funds at cheaper price is an important consideration. For instance, there are State Financial Corporation in various states which offer loans at a very low rate of interest if the entrepreneurs start their projects in the specified areas. Similarly, technocrat entrepreneurs who do not have sufficient capital to implement their projects will naturally be attracted towards these areas where they can get sufficient supply of finance.

(viii) External Economics : Sometimes industrial units are located in those centers where other industrial units are already located. It is because of the fact that transportation, warehousing, banking, communication and other services are easily available. Secondly, the raw materials may be easily available at cheaper rates. For instance, by-product of one unit may be the raw material for distilleries an other. Distilleries are located near sugar factories because molasses which is the by-product of sugar industry is the raw material for distilleries.

(ix) Personal Factor : Personal preference and prejudice of an entrepreneur may also play an important role in the choice of location. For instance, Mr. Ford started manufacturing motor cars in Detroit because it was his home town, and Lord Nuffield selected Cowley because the school in which his father was educated happened to be for sale. The success of the entrepreneur in such a location depends upon his extra personal efforts.

(x) Strategic Considerations : Strategic considerations like law and order; political stability and safety also influence location. Naturally, entrepreneurs will like to locate their units in those areas which are safe and where there are least disturbances on account of law and order problems.

(xi) Government Policy : In planned economies, the role of government policy with respect to location of industry is crucial. In India, the Central Government follows the policy of balanced regional development of the country which is necessary from the point of view of defence and social problems like slum, disparity of income and wealth and optimum use of resources. In order to implement this policy, the Government encourages industrialists to invest their money in backward areas by giving various tax incentives in the form of remission of excise duty or sales tax. Government also offers certain non-tax incentives like loan at cheaper rates, factory, sheds, etc., to attract the entrepreneurs. The Government has also announced that in future generally no license will be given to industries to be set up in metropolitan cities with a population of more than 10 lakhs and urban areas with more than 5 lakhs population as per 1971 census.

(xii) Miscellaneous Factors : Miscellaneous factors like historical incidents and attitude of the community also influence location of industries. In mug hal days, cottage industries thrived near the courts of rulers due to the patronage of State. Industrial relations atmosphere also affects the location. Facilities like housing, medical, recreation, banking and credit also attract the location of certain industrial units.

(xiii) Government Policy on Industrial Location: In a planned economy like India location of industries is an important factor in the creation of a climate for the balanced economic growth of various regions. In the absence of regulation of industrial location by the Government, industrialists are generally attracted towards the places where the industries are already developed. They do so because they will get a large number of external economies from those places. The private entrepreneurs decide the location by keeping in view the economic considerations only. They do not think in terms of social cost-benefit. This leads to the concentration of industries at particular places. There are many disadvantages of concentration of industries in particulars areas from the point of view of the society. Concentration of industries gives rise to problems of housing, transport, health and other social services. It gives rise to congestion of traffic, overcrowding and other problems also. Concentration of industries at particular places takes place at the cost of other areas. Thus, backward areas remain backward. Moreover, concentration of industries is not equitable because people living near the industries places will enjoy many benefits of industrial development including employment opportunities. People living in other areas are deprived of these benefits. Hence, Government regulation becomes necessary for the dispersal of industries to achieve balanced regional development and to avoid the problems caused by concentration.

Impact of improper location planning

A factory or a plant is the manufacturing facility of a company. A warehouse is the storage facility of a manufacturing or a distribution company. The offices of a service sector company such as a courier company, a bank, or an insurance company are its facilities. The facility location decision is very important for big business houses as well as new entrepreneurs. Wrong location of the facility may lead to a failure of the complete project. The following Figure shows the repercussions of setting up a facility without proper location planning.

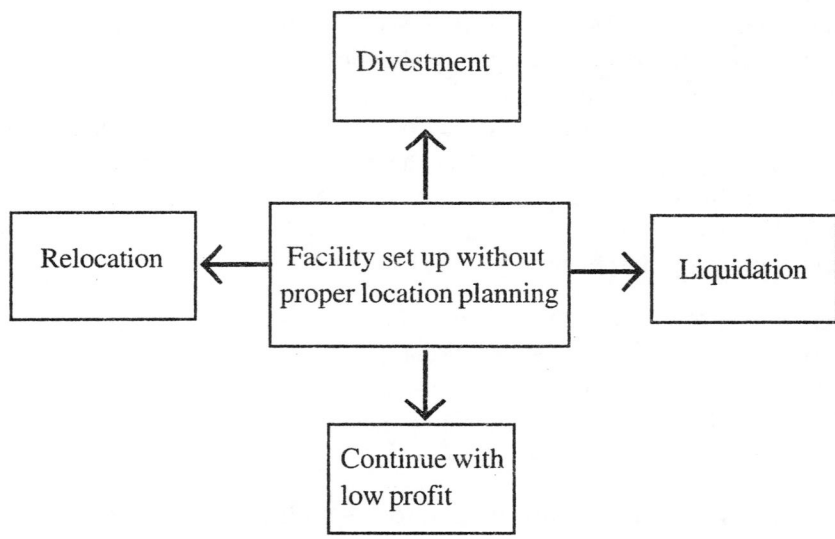

Facility without proper location planning

Sell off the facility to other companies (divestment)
- Finding buyer companies for a facility at a wrong location is difficult.
- The prices received for sell-off are usually much less than the actual investment made.
- Divestment is a time-consuming process

Relocate facility to a new location
- Only machines and equipment can be relocated, not the human resource.
- Capital expenditures such as land, buildings, etc. have to be sold, which may take a long time and the investment is blocked.
- More investment is required to purchase land, construct the building, set up machines and equipment, and hire and train new workers from scratch at the new location.

Close down the operations completely and liquidate the assets
- Liquidation of assets is most painful for any organization.
- Finding buyers and negotiating with them for different assets is tedious and time-consuming.
- The prices received for sell-off are usually much less than the actual investment made.

Continue operations at the existing location
- Inherent problems at the location become disadvantageous leading to low profit/ less market share.
- Competitors having plants at better locations always have an edge.
- In the long run, the company will have to plan another facility at the right location in order to beat competition.

2.6 TYPES OF PLANT LAYOUTS

There are three basic types of layouts that have been identified in manufacturing plants: (a) Process layout, (b) product layout, and (c) fixed-position layout. In addition, there is one hybrid that is referred to as a group technology or cellular layout, which is a combination of process and product layouts.

Process Layout

It is also called a job-shop layout or layout by function. Similar equipment or functions are grouped together, such as in a machine shop where all the lathes are in one area and all the stamping machines are in another. A part being worked on travels from one area to the next, according to the specific sequence of operations required. This type of layout is often found in high-mix, low-volume manufacturing plants that have an intermittent process.

Product Layout

It is also called a flow-shop layout. It is one in which equipment or work processes are arranged according to the progressive steps by which the product is made. If equipment is dedicated to the continual production of a narrow product line, this is usually called a *production line* or *assembly line*. Examples are the manufacture of small appliances (toasters, irons, beaters), large appliances (dishwashers, refrigerators, washing machines), electronics (computers, CD players), and automobiles.

Group Technology (GT) or Cellular Layout

It brings together dissimilar machines into work centers (or cells) to work on products that have similar shapes and processing requirements. A GT layout is similar to process layout, in that cells are designed to perform a specific set of processes, and it is similar to product layout in that the cells are dedicated to a limited range of products. Often the cell is arranged in a U-shape to allow workers to move more easily from one station to another.

Fixed-position Layout

It by virtue of its bulk or weight, the product remains stationary at one location. The manufacturing equipment is moved to the product rather than vice versa. Shipyards and construction sites are good examples of this format. Many manufacturing facilities often have a combination of two layout types. For example, a given floor may be laid out by process, while another floor may be laid out by product. It is also common to find an entire plant arranged according to general product flow (fabrication, subassembly, and final assembly), coupled with process layout within fabrication and product layout within the assembly department. Likewise, group technology is frequently found within a department that it is located according to a plant wide process-oriented layout. An operation's layout continually changes over time because the internal and external environments are dynamic. As demands change, so can layout. As technology changes, so can layout.

Facility lay-out for service

The overall goal in designing a layout for a service facility, from an operations perspective, is to minimize travel time for workers, and, often, also for customers when they are directly involved in the process. From a marketing perspective, however, the goal is usually to maximize revenues. Frequently these two goals are in conflict with each other. It is therefore management's task to identify the trade-offs that exist in designing the layout, taking both perspectives into consideration. For example, the prescription center in a pharmacy is usually located at the rear, requiring customers to walk through the store. This encourages impulse purchases of nonprescription items.

Principles of a Good Layout Manufacturing

- Straight-line Flow Pattern when possible
- Backtracking kept to a Minimum
- Predictable Production Time
- Little in-process materials storage
- Open Floor plans so everyone can see what is going on
- Bottlenecks under control
- Workstations close together
- Minimum of material handling
- Easy adjustment to changing conditions

Principles of Good Layout Face to Face Services

- Easily understood service flow pattern
- Adequate waiting facilities
- Easy communication with customers
- Customers in view of servers throughout the process
- Clear entry and exit points with adequate checkout facilities
- Customers see only what you want them to see
- Balance between waiting and service areas
- Minimum walking and material movement
- Lack of clutter
- High sales volume per square foot of service facility

2.7 METHODS OF PRODUCTION

The various methods of production are not associated with a particular volume of production. Similarly, several methods may be used at different stages of the overall production process.

Job Production

With Job production, the complete task is handled by a single worker or group of workers. Jobs can be small-scale/low technology as well as complex/high technology.

Low technology jobs: here the organisation of production is extremely simply, with the required skills and equipment easily obtainable. This method enables customer's specific requirements to be included, often as the job progresses. Examples include: hairdressers; tailoring.

High technology jobs: high technology jobs involve much greater complexity - and therefore present greater management challenge. The important ingredient in high-technology job production is project management, or project control. The essential features of good project control for a job are:

- Clear definitions of objectives - how should the job progress (milestones, dates, stages)

- Decision-making process - how are decisions taking about the needs of each process in the job, labour and other resources Examples of high technology / complex jobs: film production; large construction projects (e.g. the Millennium Dome)

Batch Production

As businesses grow and production volumes increase, it is not unusual to see the production process organised so that "**Batch methods**" can be used. Batch methods require that the work for any task is divided into parts or operations. Each operation is completed through the whole batch before the next operation is performed. By using the batch method, it is possible to achieve specialisation of labour. Capital expenditure can also be kept lower although careful planning is required to ensure that production equipment is not idle. The main aims of the batch method are, therefore, to:

- Concentrate skills (specialisation)
- Achieve high equipment utilisation

This technique is probably the most commonly used method for organising manufacture. A good example is the production of electronic instruments. Batch methods are not without their problems. There is a high probability of poor work flow, particularly if the batches are not of the optimal size or if there is a significant difference in productivity by each operation in the process. Batch methods often result in the build up of significant "work in progress" or stocks (i.e. completed batches waiting for their turn to be worked on in the next operation).

Mass Production

Mass production (also called flow production, repetitive flow production, series production, or serial production) is the production of large amounts of standardized products, including and especially on assembly lines. The concepts of mass production are applied to various kinds of products, from fluids and particulates handled in bulk (such as food, fuel, chemicals, and mined minerals) to discrete solid parts (such as fasteners) to assemblies of such parts (such as household appliances and automobiles).

Mass production is the creation of many products in a short period of time using time-saving techniques such as assembly lines and specialization. It allows a manufacturer to produce more per worker-hour, and to lower the labor cost of the end product. This in turn allows the product to be sold for a lower cost.

Mass production is the name given to the method of producing goods in large quantities at low cost per unit. But mass production, although allowing lower prices, does not have to mean low-quality production. Instead, mass-produced goods are standardized by means of precision-manufactured, interchangeable parts. The mass production process itself is characterized by mechanization to achieve high volume, elaborate organization of materials flow through various stages of manufacturing, careful supervision of quality standards, and minute division of labour.

The aims Mass production method are:

- Improved work & material flow
- Reduced need for labour skills
- Added value / completed work faster

2.8 WORLD CLASS MANUFACTURING

The concern for improving performance continuously and rapidly, in line with the increasing global competition is gathering momentum. Various performance measures provide clear insight into real problems and they, in turn, help in correcting deviations, if they exist. If a system fails to give desirable results, then the fault is not with the culture or the level of technology or labour. It is due to ineffective and incorrect performance measures used. Hence, identification and definition of right type of performance measures are to be given the top most priority.

World Class Manufacturing concept is of a recent origin. The following attributes of the World Class Manufacturing are aimed to fulfill the customer demands:

1. Products with high quality
2. Products at competitive price
3. Products with several enhanced features
4. Products in a wider variety
5. Products delivered with shorter lead times
6. Products delivered on time
7. Flexibility in fulfilling products' demand

All these performance measures are external to the manufacturing system but highly essential for the success of the company. These can be measured internally. Companies must set up their performance measures in these lines so that the product will have a high level of acceptance at customer point. The success of the company in the face of stiff competition is a direct consequence of its manufacturing function having a superior performance measurement system over its competitors. Under the World Class

Manufacturing, the company's products should have a specification closer to the customer needs than those made by any competitor, they should reach the customer error free, get delivered in a lead time faster than any other competitor, and should always be delivered at the promised due dates.

Products and service organisation are similar to each other in many ways. Manufacturing organizations not only produce goods but also provide after sales service, warranty service etc. Similarly, service organizations produce products e.g., insurance companies talk of designing new insurance schemes. Both manufacturing and service involve a transformation process in their production process, which converts various inputs into desired output, i.e., goods and services.

A modern operations manager has to focus on performance, cost minimization, delivery reliability and product quality in order to focus on customer satisfaction. Today's manufacturing operations face the daunting challenge of producing higher and higher volumes with increasing product mix, while simultaneously improving throughput, quality, compliance, and overall efficiency. Complex plans, schedules, processes, procedures and work instructions must all be executed while compliance with standards and customer requirements is demonstrated. The overall complexity of manufacturing operations management information is further increased by frequent changeovers, and the reduced proportion of manufacturing time spent in steady state operations.

2.9 NEW PRODUCT DEVELOPMENT PROCESS

In business and engineering, new product development (NPD) is the term used to describe the complete process of bringing a new product or service to market. There are two parallel paths involved in the NPD process: one involves the idea generation, product design, and detail engineering; the other involves market research and marketing analysis. Companies typically see new product development as the first stage in generating and commercializing new products within the overall strategic process of product life cycle management used to maintain or grow their market share.

The NPD process focuses on how a development project is to be structured, managed, controlled and organised. The *design process* can be viewed in the context of the NPD process as the sequence of design activities and decisions to progress from idea to detailed solution. The design process is essentially iterative and involves the definition of the problem, gathering and codification of relevant information, a divergent search for solutions, convergence on the preferred solution and detailed implementation and optimisation. It has a narrower scope than the NPD process and is not concerned with management and control issues. For practical purposes, most organisations make no distinction between the NPD process and the design process.

The new product development process consists of the following stages:

a. Ideation overview
b. Screening overview
c. Design overview
d. Design for manufacturing
e. Testing
f. Launch overview

Ideation overview

The NPD process starts with the generation of pursuable ideas. This initial phase - often referred to as the "fuzzy frontend" - is typically the most frustrating for left-brained managers who self-describe themselves as long on analytical skills, but short on creativity. In fact, though, effective new product development is a blend of creativity (creating a new world) and analysis (fitting an existing world) that maximizes potential while containing risk. The inspiration for the new product ideas can come from a driven leader (top-down) or can bubble up from trenches (bottom-up).

And while ideas can occasionally emerge from near-divine spontaneous inspiration, most mere mortals have to resort to systematic idea generation processes that range from traditional market research techniques (surveys and observation) that tend to find the "white spaces" in the existing world - to mind-stretching analyses of cultural and technological trends and scenarios that provide far-reaching directional visions of the future. Some studies have concluded that over 85% of the relevant customer input can usually be garnered from relatively small "impact" samples of 10 to 20 subjects.

Screening overview

A classic NPD question is whether success is built on the quantity of ideas (making lots of "$2 bets") or fewer, higher quality ideas ("having better at bats"). As a general rule, "more" tends to be appropriate during the ideation stage when the goal is creativity bounded only by a modicum of practicality ("innocent until proven guilty"). But, successful companies are reported to put 10 times fewer new product ideas into development per successful product as unsuccessful companies.

So, an effective NPD process is, in effect, a funnel with a large number of initial ideas sequentially pared down to the chosen few with the highest potential. The screening stage is the first tollgate in the paring process. In essence, the process of screening and prioritizing NPD ideas is a function of three factors:

(a) **Strategic attractiveness:** Does the initiative enhance the company's competitive position by leveraging existing (or prospective) strengths to capitalize on an opportunity, or neutralize a competitive or technological threat?

(b) **Financial attractiveness**: Are profits (long and short-run) sufficiently high relative to required front-end investment (ROI) when project risk is considered?

(c) **Capability to execute**: Does the company have the requisite skills and necessary resources to complete the project and support the launched product?

Design overview

The output of the screening phase is a reduced set of projects passes through to a formal design process that includes developing product specifications, selecting technologies, compiling drawings, and building prototypes. Recognizing that customer perceptions are paramount and that roughly 75-80% of a product's ultimate costs are "hard wired" in during the design phase, there are four complementary concepts that frame the design process:

The essence of **Quality Function Deployment(QFD)** is, first, to specify products in "consumer-speak" that reflects the end benefits that are most important to potential buyers, paying particular attention to quality cues, those attributes that most powerfully communicate a product's overall level of quality (e.g. the firmness of keys on a laptop pc). Engineers then translate these consumer benefits into a more technical definition of requirements. Finally, the engineering definitions are translated into very precise specifications that provide the measurements for implementing and monitoring the manufacturing process. Once the product is technically "right", the process is reversed and communications convey back to the customers that the benefits have been delivered in the product

Target costing is a formal process that attempts to mesh a proposed product's features (benefits) with a viable market price that achieves the company's profitability goals by:

(1) Determining a price point (or range of prices) for an approximate combination of features and benefits.

(2) Subtracting a desired profit from the market price to determine the maximum bearable level of costs.

(3) Iterating the product design - eliminating or reducing unnecessary attributes with costs that can't be recovered in higher prices - until the cost target is met.

(4) Revalidating the viability of the market price for the redesigned product.

Design for manufacturing

Design for manufacturing is the concurrent consideration of what a product is and how it is made, in order to insure quality, minimize costs and maximize flexibility. Narrowly defined, DFM focuses on such things as repeatable tolerances (making sure that parts are not so precisely designed that they can't be produced in mass quantities), ease of assembly (e.g. efficient sequencing of "doable" operations), and adaptability to high-speed automation (which may improve both cost and quality at high volumes). More broadly, given a growing trend towards mass customization (near infinite product variations for "segments of size one"), DFM includes:

(a)   Common components and standardized parts across products, enabling more stable forecasting (the pooling effect) and efficient management of shared inventories.

(b)   Modular platforms that include base models and a variety of add-ons that can be pre-assembled and managed "virtually".

(c)   Postponement of product differentiation until the latest possible stage in the manufacturing process (end of line customization), enabling both a high degree of standardized production and a highly customized product.

Testing

Prior to full-scale product launches, many companies put new products and their supporting marketing programs through validating tests. For example, packaged goods companies, such as P&G, traditionally test market new products in isolated geographic areas that are considered broadly representative (i.e. have characteristics common with other markets). In concept, the test markets provide a "shake out" of the actual product, allow experimentation with alternative marketing programs (e.g. different prices or different levels of advertising support), and provide results that may be projected to other markets. But, test marketing per se has become less common for three fundamental reasons:

1.   front-end market research and design methodologies have tightened the link with customers, making market responses somewhat more predictable

2.   competitors' market surveillance has become more sophisticated, alerting them to test market activity and allowing them to influence (i.e. contaminate) test market results

3.   competitors benefit from a "heads up" that may signal the need to launch a fast-follow product of their own.

Nonetheless, for high technology products, it is common to beta test radically new products. The beta tests put near-complete products (such as software) in the hands of impact users to surface any remaining bugs and establish a reference base for the product.

Launch overview

During the launch phase, there are two dominating objectives:

(a)   Secure an adequate distribution base (i.e. get intermediaries to carry the product)

(b)   Build and convert purchase intention across potential buyers.

Intermediaries are gatekeepers for new products. For upstart or unproven brands, signing up intermediaries may be a formidable challenge. For large national brands (e.g. Black & Decker), broad scale distribution support is relatively assured based on prior performance (reputation) and established account relationships. Many companies solicit intermediaries' input early-on in design process to benefit from their perspective and induce eventual "buy in". Creating and converting purchase intention typically follows the hierarchical sequence of building brand and product awareness among potential customers, communicating the product's distinctive benefits and value proposition, and informing customers when and where the product can be bought.

The level of resources (time, money, people) required to launch a product can be substantial, including dedicated sales people (to secure distribution), advertising (to build awareness and purchase intentions), promotional incentives (e.g. introductory allowances to create urgency), and merchandising support (product displays or in-store demonstrators). Accordingly, product launches can range from a "big bang" release into all markets, or sequential phasing by geographic market, channel of distribution, or customer segment. For example, a product may be launched in a confined region and then rolled out to other areas, or select intermediaries (like Wal-mart) may get initial exclusive rights to the product, or current customers may be given an early opportunity to upgrade legacy versions of the product.

Typically, a phased roll-out is most appropriate when:

1. required launch resources (e.g. ad budgets or dedicated sales people) are substantial

2. the "ramping up" of production and distribution capacity is progressive, but slow

3. time is not of the essence (e.g. competitors are not likely to be first-in to deferred markets)

4. the product must be "proven" for widespread acceptance by intermediaries and end-users.

The line between phased and big bang launches is blurring. While products may be launched in strategic phases, the time between phases is typically getting shorter (i.e. the launch cycle is faster).

SUMMARY

Products and service organisation are similar to each other in many ways. Manufacturing organizations not only produce goods but also provide after sales service, warranty service etc. Similarly, service organizations produce products e.g., insurance companies talk of designing new insurance schemes. Both

manufacturing and service involve a transformation process in their production process, which converts various inputs into desired output, i.e., goods and services. A modern operations manager has to focus on performance, cost minimization, delivery reliability and product quality in order to focus on customer satisfaction. Today's manufacturing operations face the daunting challenge of producing higher and higher volumes with increasing product mix, while simultaneously improving throughput, quality, compliance, and overall efficiency. The different methods of production include Job, Batch and Mass. The plant layout is very important based on the type of production. The different layouts are process, product, fixed position and Cellular. Production planning and control ensures all the goals and objectives of production organisation. New product development is a continuous process to sustain in the competitive environment.

REVIEW QUESTIONS

1. What is Manufacturing and Production?

2. Define Production Management and Manufacturing Management

3. What are the goals of Production management?

4. Discuss the decisions areas of Production Management

5. Explain the different methods of production.

6. What is Production, planning and control (PPC)? Discus it's functions

7. Why the facility location study is important for a business firm?

8. What are the different components of facility location planning?

9. Explain the various factors to be considered while taking the decision on facility location?

10. What are the different facility layouts available in Production Management?

11. Discuss in detail the new product development process

Chapter 3

WORK STUDY

3.1 INTRODUCTION

The pioneers in the field of work study are F.W. Taylor, F.b. Gilbreth and Lillian, M.Gilbreth. The former developed the technique of time study for determining the expected level of work performance and the later developed the technique of motion study for improving the method of doing any given work. This is the foundation based on which the modern work study stands today. Production managers strive to improve every facet of manufacturing i.e., a better product desing, improved processes, improved work methods etc., to ensure the best possible use of available resources (man-machine-material) in carrying out a specific activity. The technique of work study facilitates the same. It is a misconception that the concepts of work study are applicable only to manufacturing organisations, they are equally valid for service sector industries (like Banking, Hotel industry, Hospital Retail businesses).

Work study:

British standard Glossary defines work study as follows: "It is a generic term for those techniques, particularly method study and work measurement, which are used in the examination of human work in all its contents, and which lead systematically to the investigation of all the factors which affect the efficiency and economy of the situation being reviewed, in order to effect improvement.

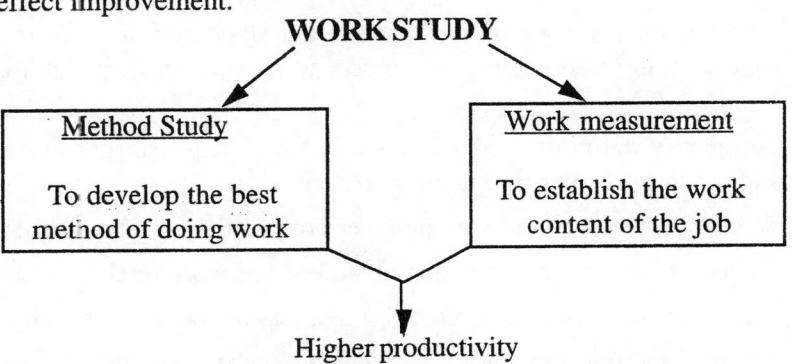

Figure: Over view of Work study

Method Study

It is the "systematic recording and critical examination of existing and proposed ways of doing work, as a means of developing and applying easier and more effective methods and reducing costs."

Work Measurement

It is the "application of techniques designed to establish the time for a qualified worker to carry out a specified job at a defined level of performance."

From the above it can be understood that work study guides us about how the jobs should be done and how long they should take.

Objectives of Work Measurement:

i). To determine the standard time required by a qualified worker to do a job.

ii). To determine man power requirements of a plant.

iii). As a basis for developing sound in centre schemes.

iv). Reliable indices for labour performance.

v). As a basis labour budgeting and budgetary control systems.

vi). Improved planning and control of activities

vii). To estimate future labour requirements and costs.

Need or Purpose of Work Measurement

i). The technique of work measurement is used to measure the time taken in the performance of an operation or a group of operations, in such a way that effective time can be separated from ineffective time. That is standard time of performing an operation and standard output level can be set.

ii). To evaluate worker's performance to set standards of performance. These standards are used to measure current worker performance in a comparative basis.

iii). To identify the most productive workers and help management better assign and organise workers to maximise output.

iv). To determine the number of employees required for performing a job.

v). To determine plant capacity at a given level of work force and equipment.

vi). It provides the basis for comparison of alternate methods of doing a job.

vii). Realistic and fair wage incentive schemes can be developed. Hence employees get more wages for more output.

The following diagram will give the different stages involved in work measurement.

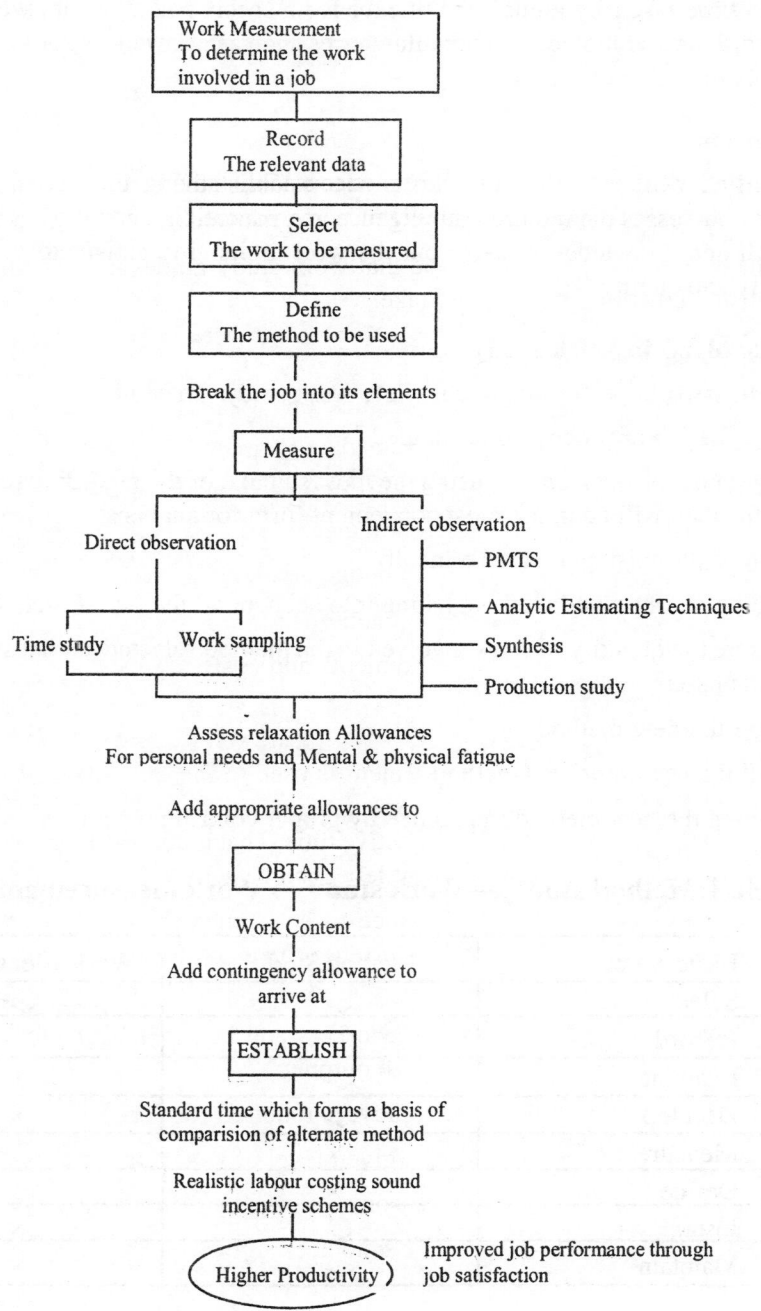

Standard Time:

It is the time taken by a qualified worker for a specific task or job, working under moderate conditions and including other allowances such as allowances for fatigue, setting of tools for job, repairing of tools etc.

Qualified worker:

A qualified worker is the one who is accepted as having the necessary physical attributes, who possesses the required intelligence and education, and who has acquired the necessary skill and knowledge to carry out the work in hand to satisfactory standards of safety, quantity and quality.

Procedure involved in work study

There are eight steps in performing a complete work study. They are:

Step 1: Select the job or process to be studied

Step 2: Record how it is performed, using the most suitable of the recording techniques, so that the data will be in the most convenient form for analysis.

Step 3: Examine the existing method critically

Step 4: Develop an improved method, taking into account all the circumstances.

Step 5: Measure the quantity of work involved in the method selected so that standard time is calculated.

Step 6: Define the new method

Step 7: Install the new improved method

Step 8: Maintain the new method in practice by proper control procedures

Table 1:Method study ← Work study → Work measurement

Sr.No	Basic Steps	Method Study	Work Measurement
1	Select	✓	✓
2	Record	✓	✓
3	Examine	✓	✓
4	Develop	✓	✕
5	Measure	✕	✓
6	Define	✕	✓
7	Install	✓	✕
8	Maintain	✓	✕

3.2 METHOD STUDY (METHOD ANALYSIS)

Method study is the systematic recording, analysis and critical examination of the methods and movements involved in the performance of existing or proposed ways of doing work, as a means of developing easier and more productive methods. It is essentially concerned with finding better ways of doing things. It contributes to improved efficiency by getting rid of unnecessary work, avoidable delays and other forms of waste. It is also known as method improvement or work improvement.

Objectives of Method Study

The method study is conducted to achieve the following objectives. They are:

i).   To critically examine the existing/proposed method of doing any job (activity)

ii). To bring improvement in working processes and procedures.

iii). To improve factory, shop and work place layout and of the design of plant and equipment.

iv). To economise human efforts and to reduce unnecessary fatigue.

v).   To improve the utilisation of resources (men-material-machines)

vi). To bring in improvement in the physical working conditions and work environment.

Area of Application

The following defects in an organisation indicate where method study is likely to bring in worth while savings.

1. Defects of layout and planning can be eliminated thus minimising excessive movement of materials and workmen.

2. Poor management of men-materials – machines results in

    i) High scrap and wastage

    ii) High operating and reprocessing costs

3. Lack of consistency in quality.

4. Existence of bottlenecks in production

5. Employees' complaints about poor working conditions, uneven distribution of workload, increasing number of accidents.

6. Excessive overtime.

Procedure involved in method study

The various steps involved in method study are as follows:

Step 1: Select the work or the job or the procedure to be studied along with the objectives to be achieved. The selection of a job depends on

i) Economic factors which include the cost of the study, the time required for the study and the associated benefits of implementing the new recommended method. It is always a trade off between the cost of the study and the profits to be earned if the new method is implemented.

ii) Technical factors and

iii) Human reactions: It is human to resist change. There can arise negative emotional reactions towards investigation and change of method among employees cooperation from the employees can be gained by educating them about the advantages of the study (investigation) and the need to continuously improve the work systems.

Step 2: Record all the relevant facts about the present method by direct observation or using any of the following recording techniques.

➤Outline process chart (or) operation process chart	It records principal operations and inspections
➤Flow process chart	They are of men, material and machine / equipment type.These charts records activities of men, materials or equipment.
➤Two handed process chart	It records activities of worker's two hands.
➤Multiple activity chart	It records activities of men/machines on a common time scale.
➤Simultaneous motion cycle (SIMO chart)	It records worker's hands, legs and other body movements on a common time scale.
➤Travel chart	It records movements of materials between departments.
➤Other charts like	Man-Machine chartMotion chartFilm analysis chart can also be used.

Diagrams & Models:

➢ Flow and string diagrams	Path of movement of men, material or equipment is recorded as diagrams.
➢ Two & three dimensional models	Layout of work-place or plant is recorded as diagrams.
➢ Cycle graphs or chrono cycle graphs	High speed, short cycle operation are recorded as diagrams.

Step 3: Examine: Critically scrutinise the recorded facts challenging everything that is being done. Each activity or job is subjected in turn to a systematic and progressive series of questions. These questions are classified as primary and secondary questions. The set of primary questions follows a well-established pattern which examine.

   i)   The purpose for which the activities are undertaken

   ii)   The place at which the activities are undertaken

   iii) The sequence in which the activities are undertaken

   iv)   The person by which the activities are undertaken

   v)   The means by which the activities are undertaken aimed at eliminating, combining and rearranging the activities involved in a job.

At the secondary stage, the questions are meant to seek possible alternatives which are practicable and preferable as a means of improvement. That is the method study manager questions about what else can be done to improve the present method.

Step 4: Develop several alternatives to the existing method and select the best method. The following factors need to be considered while evaluating alternatives to select the best method.

   a)   Expected savings in time and cost.

   b)   Acceptance of the new method by production planning and control, quality control and sales departments.

   c)   Acceptance of the new method by the trade unions and employees of the organisation.

   d)   Feasibility of implementation

   e)   Short term and long term implications of the alternative.

Step 5: Install: A typical installation of the improved method can be divided into five stages. They are

   a)   Gaining acceptance of the change by the departmental supervision.

   b)   Gaining approval of the change by the management

c) Gaining acceptance of the change by the workers involved and their representatives

d) Restrain the workers to operate the new methods

e) Maintaining close contact with the progress of the job until satisfied that it is running as intended.

Step 6: Maintain: To be maintained, a method must first be defined clearly. Ensure that the new installed method is functioning well in its specified form. Proper control procedures are to be used to ensure that operators are not slipping back into old methods, or introducing elements not allowed for unless there is a valid reason. There should be periodic checks and verification at regular intervals to see that the new method is practised to achieve the desired objectives.

3.3 CONCEPT OF QUALITY

Introduction

Nowadays, we are all victims of quality failures daily, such as late trains and aero planes, leaking car-door seals and prematurely expiring light bulbs. The consumer is invariably the loser as the real costs of a quality failure may be much more than the value of the defective good or service. Customers are becoming increasingly intolerant of poor service, late deliveries, unreliable goods, shoddy workmanship and the like. They are exerting control over the suppliers by preferring to buy from alternative sources. For example, the US customers for automobiles showed sharp preference for Japanese cars in the US Automobile market. The reputation of Japanese car manufacturers for the reliability and 'value for money' for their cars posed a serious threat to their western competitors.

Evolution of Quality Management

In the early 1900s, F.W. Taylor, the 'Father of Scientific Management', emphasized on quality by including product inspection and gauging in his list of fundamental areas of manufacturing management. G.S. Radford's contributions were notions of involving quality consideration early in the product design stage and linking together high quality, increased productivity and lower costs. In 1924, W.Shewhart introduced statistical control charts to monitor production. Around 1930, H.F.Dodge and H.G.Romig introduced tables for acceptance sampling. World War II caused a dramatic increase in emphasis on quality control. Soon after, US Universities started training engineers in the use of statistical sampling techniques and professional quality organizations such as American Society for Quality Control started emerging in the US. During the 1950s, the quality movement evolved into quality assurance. W.Edward Deming introduced Statistical Quality control (SQC) methods to Japanese manufacturers to help them to rebuild their manufacturing base and to enable them to compete in the world markets.

At about the same time, Joseph Juran began his 'cost of quality' approach, emphasizing accurate and complete identification and measurement of costs of quality. In the mid 1950s, Armand Fiegen Baum proposed total quality control, which enlarged the focus of quality control. During the 1960s, Philip Crosby, who was the champion of "Zero defects" concept focused on employee motivation and awareness. In the late 1970s there was dramatic shift from quality assurance to a strategic approach to quality. The 'reactive' approach of finding and correcting defects from recurring altogether. This new strategic approach closely linked quality to productivity and profits. In addition, this approach placed greater emphasis on consumer satisfaction and involved all levels of management as well as workers in a continuing effort to increase quality.

Quality-what it stands for?

Q: Quest for excellence

U: Understanding customer's needs

A: Action to achieve customer's appreciation

L: Leadership-determination to be a leader

I : Involving all people

T: Team spirit to work for a common goal and

Y: Yardstick to measure progress.

Quality definitions

"Quality" is defined as:

a) "The ability of a product or service to meet customer needs".

b) "The totality of features and characteristics of a product or service that bears on its ability to satisfy stated or implied needs" definition adopted by the American Society for Quality".

c) "Meeting or exceeding customer requirements now and in the future". This means that the product or service is fit for customer's use. Fitness for use is related to benefits received by the customer and to ensure customer satisfaction.

d) W.Edward Deming, a leading quality guru called quality as "Continuous improvement". Another expert, Joseph M.Juran, speaks of quality as "fit for use" while Philip Crosby uses the phrase "conformance to requirements". Americans speak of "Value received for dollars spent", while Europeans emphasize quality engineered into their goods. Kaoru Ishikawa, another quality guru, thought in terms of products "most economical, most useful and always satisfactory to the consumer"

e) New thinking about 'quality'.

Old Quality is		New Quality is
About products	↔	About organizations
Technical	↔	Strategic
For inspectors	↔	For every one
Led by experts	↔	Led by management
High grade	↔	The appropriate grade
About control	↔	About improvement
"Little 'q'"	↔	"Big 'Q'"

Dimensions of quality

As customers evaluate quality of a product or service, they consider different aspects or dimensions of the product or service. Below table 1.1 describes some of the dimensions of quality that customers use to evaluate quality.

Table Some dimensions of product quality

1.	Performance	How well the product or service performs the customer's intended use. For example, the speed of a laser printer.
2	Features	The special characteristics that appeal to customers. For example, power steering and central locking system of an automobile.
3.	Reliability	The likelihood of breakdown, malfunction or the need for repairs
4	Serviceability	The speed, cost and convenience of repairs and maintenance.
5	Durability	The length of time or amount of use before needing to be repaired or replaced.
6	Appearances	The effect on human senses-the look, feel, taste, smell or sound
7	Customer service	The treatment received by customers before, during and after the sale.
8	Safety	How well the product protects users before, during and

Dimensions of service quality

a) Reliability-consistency of performer and dependability

b) Responsiveness-willingness or readiness to provide service, timeliness

c) Competence-possession of skills and knowledge required to perform the service

d) Access-approachability and ease of contact

e) Courtesy-politeness, respect, consideration for property, clean and neat appearance

f) Communication educating and informing customers in language they can understand, listening to customers.

g) Credibility-trustworthiness, belief, having customer's best interest at heart

h) Understanding-making an effort to understand the customer's needs, learning the specific requirements, providing individualized attention, and recognizing the regular customers.

i) Security-freedom from danger, risk or doubt.

j) Tangibles- the physical evidence of service (facilities, tools and equipment).

Quality Tree

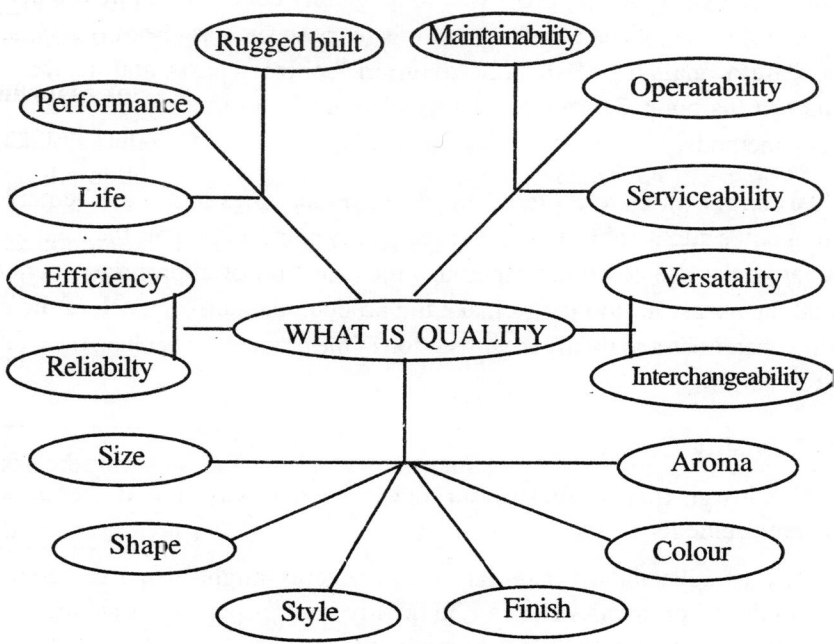

Benefits of Quality to a Firm

1. It gives a positive company image.
2. It improves competitive ability both nationally and internationally
3. It increases market share, which translates into improved profits.
4. Overall, it reduces costs, which also translates into improved profits.
5. It reduces or eliminates product liability problems, avoiding unnecessary costs.
6. It creates an atmosphere for high employee morale, which improves productivity.

Quality control

The purpose of quality control is to assure that processes are performing in an acceptable manner. This is accomplished by monitoring the process output using statistical techniques. If the results are acceptable, no further action is required. If not, corrective action is called for. The best companies emphasize designing quality into the process, thereby greatly reducing the need for inspection or control efforts. The ultimate goal of a firm is to totally avoid inspection activities and process control activities by achieving an inherent level of quality that is sufficiently high.

For analysis and improving process quality, quality control methods are used. There are seven time-tested established methods for this purpose such as check sheets, bar charts, histograms, Pareto analysis, fish bone diagram, control charts and scatter diagram. W.A.Shewhart in his book Control of Quality of Manufactured Product (1931) first used some of these methods.

Quality control refers to all those functions or activities that must be performed to fulfill the company's quality objectives. Hence, quality control involves the establishment of quality standards, the use of proper materials, the selection of appropriate manufacturing processes and the necessary tooling to make the product, the performance of the necessary manufacturing operations and finally the inspection of the product to check on the conformance with the specifications.

Functions of Quality Control

☆ To design the product or service in such a way that it meets customers requirements.

☆ Use of substandard material or components might effect the quality of the produced products. Hence, the quality control personnel should see that the purchased materials, parts, components, etc. are of standard quality.

☆ To identify and provide information on causes of variations in production process, so that corrective action is taken.

☆ To see that the produced product or service meets safety conditions. Especially in case of electrical, electronic and perishable products.

☆ To reduce the proportion of scrap, wastage & spoilage during the process.

☆ To provide satisfactory product support services i.e., after sales service.

☆ To make the employees quality conscious by fixing their responsibility at various stages of production.

☆ To prevent rather than detect defective items to be produced.

Quality of a product is to be controlled at various stages of production, namely

i) At the design stage

ii) At the purchasing (procurement of raw materials, components, parts, tools, equipments, etc.) stage.

iii) At the production stage, that is inspect test work in process or the service while it is being delivered.

iv) After the product is sold in terms of product – support services (After sales service).

Benefits of quality control

An effective quality control programme if implemented, provides the following benefits:-

1) Minimum scrap, rework and other losses.

2) Reduced cost of material and labour.

3) Uniformity of quality and reliability of products, which increases sales turnover.

4) Reduced variability.

5) Reduced inspection costs.

6) Reduced customer complaints.

7) Better utilization of resources.

8) Higher productivity and improved profits.

Approaches to Quality Control

There are three aspects involved in any quality control programme. They are :

1) **Engineering** : Engineering deals with the creation and development of a product. It is also concerned with the concepts of quality evaluation, then identifying the causes of defects and then rectifying substandard products.

2) **Statistical** : Statistical knowledge helps to build an information system, which applies quantitative techniques to determine how far the product conforms to the standards of quality and precision.

3) **Managerial** : The techniques of engineering and statistics have to be integrated by the policies and practices of the management. It is the management who creates and nurtures quality conscious climate in the organisation.

3.4   STATISTICAL QUALITY CONTROL(SQC)

The application of statistical techniques to control quality. The term "statistical process control" is often used interchangeably with "statistical quality control," although statistical quality control includes acceptance sampling as well as statistical process control.

Statistical Quality Control (S.Q.C) aims at achieving the target of conformance of the end product to the standards and expectations laid down by the customers. S.Q.C is the application of quantitative techniques to determine how far the product conforms to the standards of quality and precision and to what extent its quality deviates from the standard quality. In other words, it is a simple statistical method for determining the extent to which quality goals are being met without necessarily checking every item produced and for indicating whether or not the variations, =which occur are exceeding normal expectations. SQC enables us to decide whether to accept or reject a particular product.

Benefits of SQC:

- Easy to identify operators that are producing defects and may require additional training.
- Accurately reports defects at the operator, cut, job and style level.
- Defect analysis in either summary or detail versions.
- Up-to-the-minute operator accountability for quick and accurate repair control.
- Improved quality levels within the plant and reduced expense involved in reworking garments.

Significantly reduced cost and administrative effort required to perform SQC and Quality Auditing functions within the factory.

The following figure shows various techniques used for S Q C.

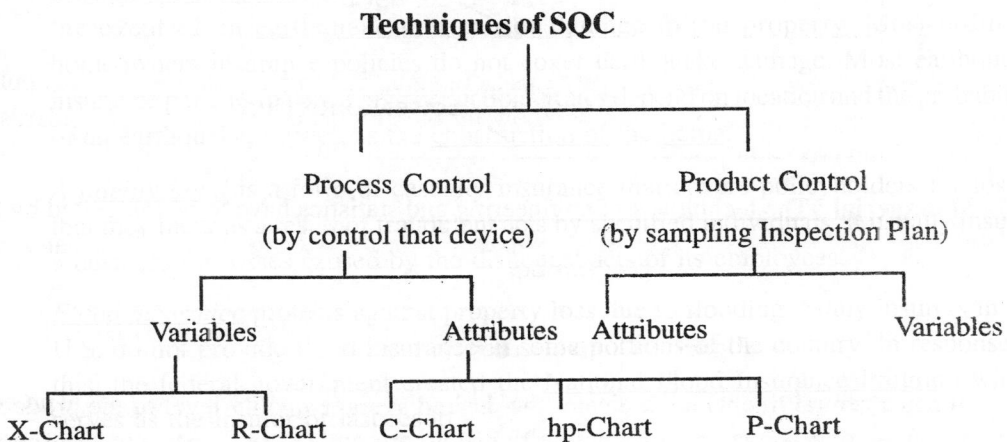

Process control is used during production while the product is being made. The decision in this case is whether to continue the process or to stop production and look for an assignable cause of defects, which could be attributed to materials, operators or the machines. Whereas acceptance sampling (product control) applies to lot inspection where a decision to accept or reject a lot of material is made on the basis of a random sample drawn from the lot. This type of inspection is done after production is completed. Acceptance sampling is defined as taking one or more samples at random from a lot of items, inspecting each of the items in the samples, and deciding on the basis of the inspection results whether to accept or reject the entire lot.

Control charts

A control chart is a graphical representation of an on going process for its quality. The quality is a measurable character. A control chart for mean($\bar{x}$ chart) can help in assessing whether the average of the process is in control or not. A control chart for Range(R chart) can help in assessing whether the variability or the spread of the process is in control or not. A typical control chart is show in figure

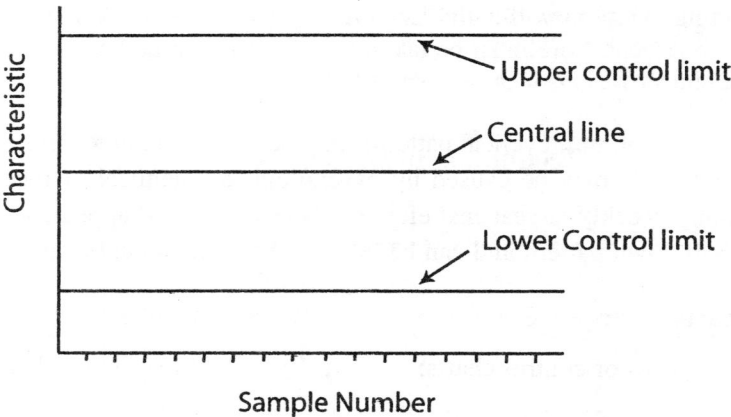

Figure : Control chart

It has a central line which indicates the desired average quality level of the product. The two lines, one above and one below this line, are called the *upper* and the *lower control limits,* respectively. These limits are established to assist in judging the significance of the variation in the quality of the product. It may be noted that the control limits are different from the *specification limits.* Whereas the specification limits refer to the quality characteristic of an *individual unit* of the product, the control limits are used to evaluate the variations in quality from sample to sample.

Once the control limits are established, samples of units of the output are examined for quality and the results of each one plotted on the chart. When a process is in control, there occurs a normal pattern of variation so that (a) about two-thirds of the sample points are near the central line, (b) some of the points are closer to the control limits, (c) the points are located back and forth across the central line, (d) the points are balanced on both sides of the line, and (e) no points lie beyond the control limits.

On the other hand, an out-of-control situation includes the following:

(a)   Point(s) outside: A point beyond either of the control limits is indicative of an external influence-the presence of an assignable cause.

(b)   Change or jump in level: Sometimes a change in the level occurs even though no points fall outside the control limits. This change can be observed when successive plotted points are on one side with respect to the central line but are still within the control limits.

(c)   Trend or steady change in level: At times, a steady progressive change in the plotted points may be observed. This is called a trend and may be caused by machine deterioration or tool wear. Care must be taken to correct the trend before it goes too far.

(d)   Recurring cycles: Sometimes, cyclical patterns may be observed in the points plotted on a control chart. This may be caused by psychological, chemical or mechanical reasons, or by daily, weekly or seasonal effects. These make their appearance on the chart by an up and down pattern and can be taken to be an assignable variation.

Types of control charts

Basically, there are two types of control charts:

     (a)   control charts for variables, and

     (b)   control charts for attributes

This classification is based on the particular characteristic of interest. If the quality characteristic under consideration is one which can be measured in quantitative terms on a continuous scale of measurement then the control charts in respect of it would be called *control charts for variable*. The quality dimensions using variable control charts include characteristics like length, width, depth, tensile strength, thickness, elasticity, moisture content etc.

On the other hand, if the characteristic cannot be measured but, instead, the items can be classified as being either defective or non-defective (for example the picture tubes used in TV sets can be either working or defective), or if the number of defects in an item may be known (for example, the number of weaving defects in a hundred-metre cloth length, airholes in glass bottles, knots and other defects in lumber), we shall have *control charts for attributes*.

We shall now consider the method of construction of the control charts, and their interpretation.

Control Charts for Variables

The construction of control charts depends upon the given information. In this context there are two possibilities. One is when the standards are given and it is required to determine whether or not the observed quality characteristic differs from sample to sample by an amount greater than the expected difference due to the operation of chance factor alone.

(a) **When standards are given** (i) **Control Chart of Mean,** $\overline{X}$ - chart: If μ and σ be the mean and standard deviation of the population from which the random samples of size n are drawn, then we have,

Central Line, $CL = \mu$

Upper Control Limit, $UCL_{\overline{x}} = \mu + \dfrac{3\sigma}{\sqrt{n}}$

Lower control limit, $LCL_{\overline{x}} = \mu - \dfrac{3\sigma}{\sqrt{n}}$

In addition to the control limits, warning limits, which are taken as a warning that the process might have gone out of control, and are determined by 1.96 distance on either side can also be shown in the $\overline{X}$ - chart. Thus, we have

Upper Warning Limit, $UWL_{\overline{x}} = \mu + \dfrac{1.96\sigma}{\sqrt{n}}$

Lower Warning Limit, $LWL_{\overline{x}} = \mu - \dfrac{1.96\sigma}{\sqrt{n}}$

Generally, the control charts show only the control limits.

Example 1

In the production of an item, the process is said to be under control if the diameters have a mean of 3.5inches and a standard deviation of 0.05inches. Construct a control chart for the mean of random samples of size (a) 10, and (b) 20, showing the warning and the control limits on the graph paper.

We are given that $\mu = 3.5$inches and $\sigma = 0.05$ inches.

(a) When $n = 10$

Central Line, $CL = 3.5$inches

Upper Control Limit, $UCL_{\overline{x}} = 3.5 + \dfrac{3 \times 0.05}{\sqrt{10}}$

$$= 3.5 + 0.047 = 3.547$$

Lower control Limit, $LCL_{\overline{x}} = 3.5 - \dfrac{3 \times 0.05}{\sqrt{10}}$

$$= 3.5 - 0.047 = 3.453 \text{ inches}$$

Upper warning Limit $\text{UWL}_{\bar{x}} = 3.5 + \dfrac{1.96 \times 0.05}{\sqrt{10}}$

$$= 3.5 + 0.03 = 3.53 \text{ inches}$$

Lower Warning Limit, $\text{LWL}_{\bar{x}} = 3.5 - \dfrac{1.96 \times 0.05}{\sqrt{10}}$

$$= 3.5 - 0.03 = 3.47 \text{ inches}$$

The control chart is show in figure

(b)   When $n = 20$

$$\text{UCL}_{\bar{x}} = 3.5 + \frac{3 \times 0.05}{\sqrt{20}}$$

$$= 3.5 + 0.034 = 3.534 \text{ inches}$$

$$\text{LCL}_{\bar{x}} = 3.5 - \frac{3 \times 0.05}{\sqrt{20}}$$

$$= 3.5 - 0.034 = 3.466 \text{ inches}$$

$$\text{UWL}_{\bar{x}} = 3.5 \frac{1.96 \times 0.05}{\sqrt{20}}$$

$$= 3.5 - 0.022 = 3.478 \text{ inches}$$

The control and warning limits are shown in the figure

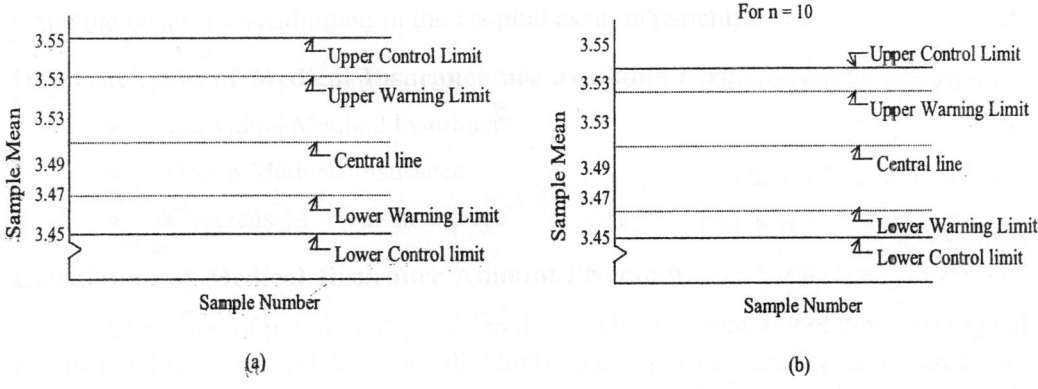

(a)   (b)

Figure : Control Chart for Mean

It is clear that for a given μ and σ, the control and warning limits are dependent on the sample size. As the sample size increases, the control limits become closer to the central line, which makes the control chart more sensitive to small variations in the process average.

(ii)   **The R-chart** : The construction of R-chart, when the population standard deviation σ is known, follows:

$$CL = d_2\sigma$$
$$UCL_R = d_2\sigma + 3d_3\sigma$$
$$LCL_R = d_2\sigma - 3d_3\sigma$$

wherein d_2 and d_3 values can be obtained from the table given at page 3.39.

It may be mentioned here that whenever a lower control limit for a range chart is obtained as negative, it shall be taken to be zero.

Example 2

Draw R-chart for the data given in example 1

(a) When $n = 10$

For $n = 10$, $d_2 = 3.078$ and $d_3 = 0.797$

Thus, CL $= 3.078 \times 0.05 = 0.1539$;

$UCL_R = 0.1539 + 3 \; 0.797 \times 0.05$

$= 0.1539 + 0.1196 = 0.2735$

$LCL_R \quad = 0.1539 - 3 \times 0.797 \times 0.05$

$= 0.1539 - 0.1196 = 0.0343$

The control chart corresponding to these values is given in figure

(b) when $n = 20$

For $n = 20$, $d_2 = 3.735$, and $d_3 = 0.729$.

CL $= 3.735 \times 0.05 = 0.18675$

$UCL_R = 0.18675 + 3 \times 0.729 \times 0.05$

$= 0.18675 + 0.10935 = 0.2961$

$LCL_R \quad = 0.18675 - 3 \times 0.729 \times 0.05$

$= 0.18675 - 0.10935 = 0.0774$

Figure contains the control chart.

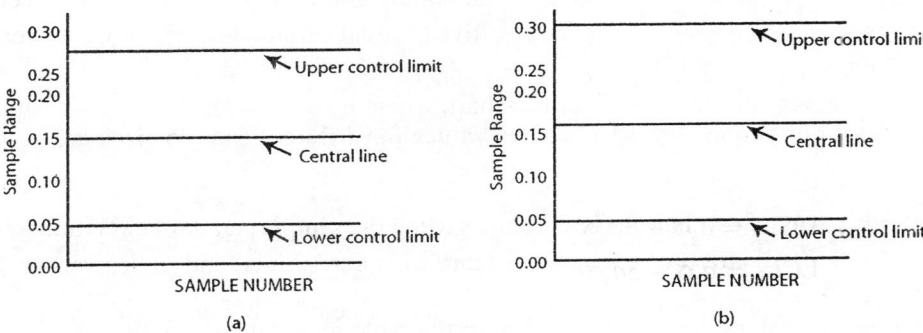

(a)   (b)

(b) **When standards are not given**

(i) Control Chart for Mean, $\overline{X}$ - chart: When the specifications are not given, then μ is estimated by $\overline{\overline{X}}$, the overall mean of the sample means which are taken for the determination of central line and the control limits. The central line and the control limits are determined as follows.

The central lines is given by $\overline{\overline{X}}$, obtained as follows:

$$\overline{\overline{X}} = \sum \overline{X}_i / k, \qquad i = 1, 2, ...k.$$

where $\overline{X}_i$ is the arithmetic mean of the ith sample.

The value of σ not being given, its value is estimated by $\overline{R} / d_2$, in which $\overline{R}$ is defined as

$$\overline{R} = \sum R_i / k, \qquad i = 1, 2, ...k.$$

where R_i is the range of the ith sample, and d_2 is a factor whose value is based on the sample size n. The values of d_2 for different sample sizes are given in the table.

Having obtained the value of $\overline{R}$, the control limits are determined as follows:

$$\mathrm{UCL}_{\overline{x}} = \overline{\overline{X}} + \frac{3\overline{R}}{d_2 \sqrt{n}}$$

$$\mathrm{LCL}_{\overline{x}} = \overline{\overline{X}} - \frac{3\overline{R}}{d_2 \sqrt{n}}$$

The control limits can be found in a more convenient and direct way as:

$$UCL_{\bar{x}} = \bar{\bar{X}} + A_2\bar{R} \quad \text{and}$$

$$LCL_{\bar{x}} = \bar{\bar{X}} - A_2\bar{R}$$

in which A_2 is defined as $3/d_2 \sqrt{n}$ and its values for different sample sizes are given in Table.

Another way of estimating the σ value is using the sample standard deviations, s. For this, the standard deviation of each of the samples is determined and their average $\bar{s}$, is obtained. The estimate of σ is given by $\bar{s}/c_2$, the value of c_2 being read from the table, keeping in mind the sample size n. The central line and control limits would be:

$$CL \quad = \bar{\bar{X}}$$

$$UCL_{\bar{x}} = \bar{\bar{X}} + \frac{3\bar{s}}{c_2\sqrt{n}}$$

$$LCL_{\bar{x}} = \bar{\bar{X}} - \frac{3\bar{s}}{c_2\sqrt{n}}$$

And, as before, 1.96 would be substituted for 3, if warning limits are desired.

(ii)   **Control Chart for Range, R-chart**: When the population standard deviation σ is not known, we estimate it using the sample data on ranges, as has been mentioned earlier. The range chart is prepared as follows.

$$CL : \bar{R} = \Sigma R_i / k$$

$$UCL_R = \bar{R} + \frac{3d_3\bar{R}}{d_2}$$

$$= \bar{R}\left[1 + \frac{3d_3}{d_2}\right] = \bar{R}D_4$$

$$LCL_R = \bar{R} = \frac{3d_3\bar{R}}{d_2}$$

$$= \bar{R}\left[1 - \frac{3d_3}{d_2}\right] = \bar{R}D_3 \,.$$

Values of D_3 and D_4 can be obtained from the table B8 in appendix B, based on the sample size n.

Example 3

Using the following data relating to 12 samples of 5 items each, calculate the control limits for the mean and the range charts. Also plot the values on them.

Dimensions (in cms) of items

1	2	3	4	5	6	7	8	9	10	11	12
1.04	0.98	0.97	1.04	1.04	1.03	1.00	1.00	0.99	0.96	0.93	1.05
0.98	0.98	0.99	1.02	1.02	1.01	1.02	1.01	1.02	0.95	0.98	1.05
0.99	0.98	1.01	1.01	1.01	0.98	0.97	0.99	1.03	1.02	0.99	0.97
1.00	1.03	0.95	1.00	1.00	1.01	0.98	0.99	1.01	1.03	1.04	1.02
1.01	1.01	0.97	1.00	1.00	1.01	0.99	0.95	0.97	1.01	1.04	0.99

Table Determination of Control Limits

1	2	3	4	5	6	7	8	9	10	11	12
1.04	0.98	0.97	1.04	1.04	1.03	1.00	1.00	0.99	0.96	0.93	1.05
0.98	0.98	0.99	1.02	1.02	1.01	1.02	1.01	1.02	0.95	0.98	1.05
0.99	0.98	1.01	1.01	1.01	0.97	0.98	0.99	1.03	1.02	0.99	0.97
1.00	1.03	0.95	1.00	1.00	0.98	1.01	0.99	1.01	1.03	1.04	1.02
1.01	1.01	0.97	1.00	1.00	0.99	1.01	0.95	0.97	1.01	1.04	0.99
Total											
5.02	4.98	5.07	4.89	5.07	4.98	5.02	4.94	5.02	4.97	4.98	5.08

From the table, we have

$$\overline{\overline{X}} = \Sigma \overline{X}_i / k \quad = \quad 12.004 / 12 = 1.0003;$$

$$\overline{R} = \Sigma R_i / k \quad = \quad 0.75 / 12 = 0.0625; \text{ and}$$

$$\overline{s} = \Sigma s_i / k \quad = \quad 0.2791/12 = 0.02326$$

(a)　　For $\overline{X}$-chart

$$CL = \overline{\overline{X}} = 1.0003$$

$$UCL_{\bar{x}} = \overline{\overline{X}} + \frac{3\overline{R}}{d_2 \sqrt{n}}$$

$$= 1.0003 + \frac{3 \times 0.0625}{2.326 \times \sqrt{5}} \text{ (since for } n = 5, d_2 \text{ equals } 2.326)$$

$$= 1.0364$$

$$\text{LCL}_{\bar{x}} = \bar{\bar{X}} - \frac{3\bar{R}}{d_2 \sqrt{n}}$$

$$= 1.0003 - \frac{3 \times 0.0625}{2.326 \times \sqrt{5}} = 0.9642$$

Note: The control limits can also be determined using the factors A_2 and c_2.

i)   For $n = 5$, $A_2 = 0.577$

thus, the control limits would be $\bar{\bar{X}} \pm A_2 \bar{R}$

$$= 1.0003 \pm 0.577 \times 0.0625$$
$$= 0.9642 \text{ and } 1.0364$$

$\bar{X}$	1.004	0.996	1.014	0.978	1.014	0.996	1.004	0.988	1.004	0.994	0.996	1.016
R	0.06	0.05	0.06	0.06	0.03	0.06	0.04	0.06	0.06	0.08	0.11	0.08
S	.0206	.0206	.0196	.0204	.0150	.0215	.0136	.0204	.0215	.0326	.0413	.0320

The $\bar{X}$-charts is shown in figure 3.13 It is clear that since all the points are within the control limits, the process is evidently in control in respect of the average quality level.

(b) For R-chart

$$\text{CL} = \bar{R} = 0.0625$$
For $n = 5$, $d_3 = 0.864$. Thus,

$$\text{UCL}_R = \bar{R} + \frac{3d_3\bar{R}}{d_2}$$

$$= 0.0625 + \frac{3 \times 0.864 \times 0.0625}{2.326}$$
$$= 0.0625 + 0.0696 = 0.1321$$

$$\text{LCL}_R = \bar{R} - \frac{3d_3\bar{R}}{d_2}$$

$$= 0.0625 - \frac{3 \times 0.864 \times 0.0625}{2.326}$$

$$= 0.0625 - 0.0696 = -0.0071 = 0 \text{ (being netative)}$$

The control limits can be obtained using D_3 and D_4 also. For $n = 5$, $D_3 = 0$ and $D_4 = 2.115$

Accordingly, $UCL_R = D_4 \overline{R} = 2.115 \times 0.0625 = 0.1321$ and

$$LCL_R = D_3 \overline{R} = 0 \times 0.0625 = 0$$

The control chart in respect of range is shown in figure

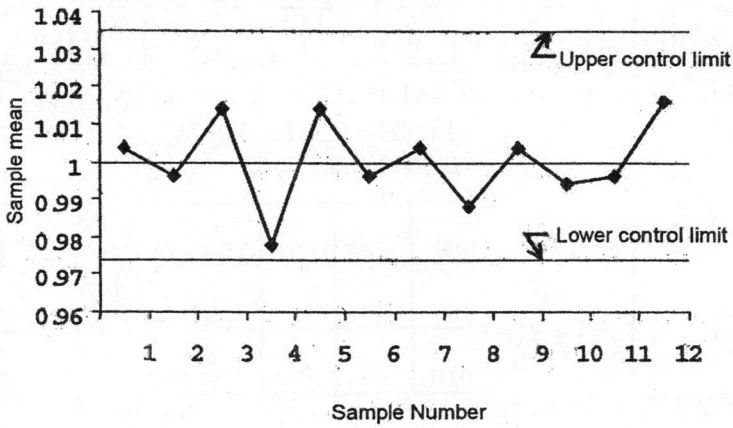

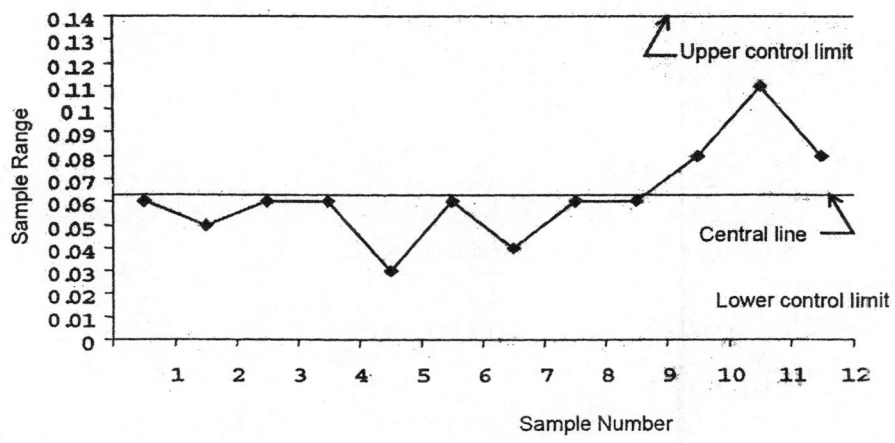

Comment: All the points in $\overline{X}$ Chart are given within the control. All the points in the R Chart are also within the control limits. Hence we can conclude that the process is in control with respect to variability.

Example 4

The following data given readings for 10 samples of size 8 each in the production of a certain component

Sample:	1	2	3	4	5	6	7	8	9	10
Mean:	5.4	5.1	5.4	4.9	5.2	4.7	5.1	5.0	5.0	5.2
Range:	0.4	0.7	0.7	0.8	0.9	0.6	0.5	0.6	0.7	0.6

Draw the control charts for mean and range, and point out which samples, if any, are out of limits.

For $\overline{X}$ chart

$$CL = \overline{X} = \sum \overline{X}_i / k \quad = 51/10 = 5.1$$

$$UCL_{\bar{x}} = \overline{\overline{X}} + \frac{3\overline{R}}{d_2\sqrt{n}}$$

For $n = 8$, since $d_2 = 2.847$, and further because $\overline{R} = \sum R_i / k = 6.5 / 10 = 0.65$, we have

$$UCL_{\bar{x}} = 5.1 + \frac{3 \times 0.65}{2.847 \times \sqrt{8}} = 5.1 + 0.2422 = 5.3422$$

$$LCL_{\bar{x}} = \overline{\overline{X}} - \frac{3\overline{R}}{d_2\sqrt{n}}$$

$$= 5.1 - \frac{3 \times 0.65}{2.847 \times \sqrt{8}}$$

$$= 5.1 - 0.2422 = 4.8578$$

For Range – chart

$$CL = \overline{R} = 0.65$$

$$UCL_R = \overline{R}D_4$$

$$= 0.65 \times 1.864 = 1.2116$$

$$LCL_R = \overline{R}D_3$$
$$= 0.65 \times 0.136 = 0.0884$$

[From the table, $D_3 = 0.136$ and $D_4 = 1.864$, for $n = 8$]
(given in page 3.39)

Samples 1, 3 and 6 in the mean chart are beyond the control limits in this case.

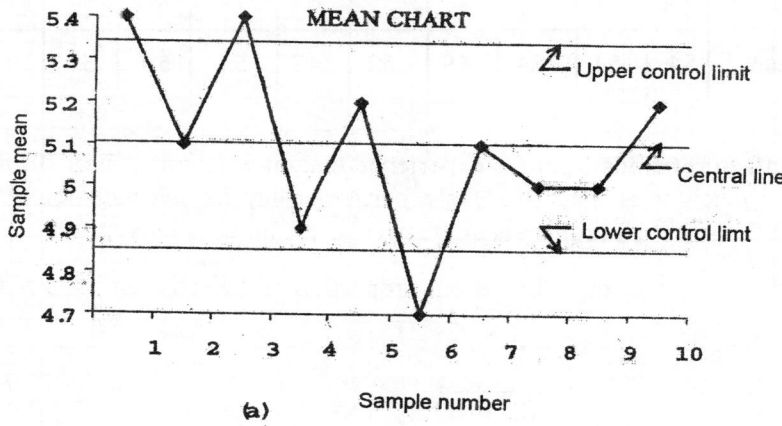

(a)

Control Charts for Attributes

There are two different types of control charts for attributes, which are based on the distinction between defectives and defects. Whereas a defective is a piece of product that in some way fails to be within the tolerances established for critical quality characteristics, each failure to meet specification is a defect, making it possible to have one or more defects in any defectives. There are two control charts for defectives; the p-chart, for the proportion of defectives in the sample, and the np-chart, for the number of defectives. They are based on the binomial distribution.

The c-chart is the control chart for the number of defects in a unit and is based on the poisson distribution. We discuss these charts in turn now.

(a) **p-chart** This is drawn on the basis of the proportion defectives in the lots. For this chart, the central line is determined by the proportion of defectives found generally in a lot, from the past experience. If the information about different samples is given, then we find the average proportion of the defectives in all samples taken together $\overline{p}$. The control limits are then determined by 3-sigma distances as follows:

$$\overline{p} \pm 3\sqrt{\frac{\overline{p}(1-\overline{p})}{n}}$$

when n is the sample size.

Of course, if information from past records is available and if p is the average defectives proportion, the limits would be given by

$$p \pm 3\sqrt{\frac{pq}{n}}$$

in which $q = 1 - p$.

Example 5

A manufacturer finds from his experience that on an average 1 in 10 of the items produced by a machine is defective. On a particular day he selects a lot of 100 items randomly and finds that 20 of them are defective. Is the process in control?

According to the given information, proportion of defective units, $p = 1/10 = 0.1$. Thus,

$$CL = 0.1$$

$$UCL_p = 0.1 + 3\sqrt{\frac{0.1 \times 0.9}{100}}$$

$$= 0.1 + 0.09 = 0.19$$

$$LCL_p = 0.1 - 3\sqrt{\frac{0.1 \times 0.9}{100}}$$

$$= 0.1 - 0.09 = 0.01$$

For the observed sample, since we have $p = 20 / 100 = 0.20$, which is beyond the UCL_p, the process in all probability is not control.

(b)   *np*-**chart:** It is similar to the *p*-chart except that the focus is on the number of defectives found in the different samples. We know that with the sample size n and the proportion of defectives p, the average number of defectives would be np. For the *np*-chart, the average number of defectives usually found (from the past records) or the average number of defectives in all samples taken together, determines the central line. The control limits are given by

$$n\overline{p} \pm 3\sqrt{(n\overline{p}(1-\overline{p}))}$$

Example 6

In the following table are given the number of defectives found on 24 consecutive production days in daily samples of 200 items. Draw (a) an *np*- chart, and (b) a *p*-chart. Which points fall outside the control limits?

Production Day	1	2	3	4	5	6	7	8	9	10	11	12
No of Defectives	10	5	10	12	11	9	19	4	12	27	25	9
Production Day	13	14	15	16	17	18	19	20	21	22	23	24
No of Defectives	12	15	8	14	10	4	11	11	26	3	10	11

Here,

Total number of units examined =   No of samples × sample size

$\qquad\qquad\qquad\qquad\qquad\quad =$ 24 × 200 = 4800

Total number of units defective =   288

∴ Average proportion of defectives,

$$\bar{p} = \frac{\text{No of defectives}}{\text{No of units}} = \frac{288}{4800} = 0.06$$

(a)   *np*-chart

$$CL = n\bar{p} = 200 \times 0.06 = 12$$

Control Limits $= n\bar{p} \pm 3\sqrt{n\bar{p}(1-\bar{p})}$

$$= 12 \pm 3\sqrt{200 \times 0.06 \times 0.94}$$

$$= 1.92 \text{ and } 22.08$$

The given data and the control limits are given in figure

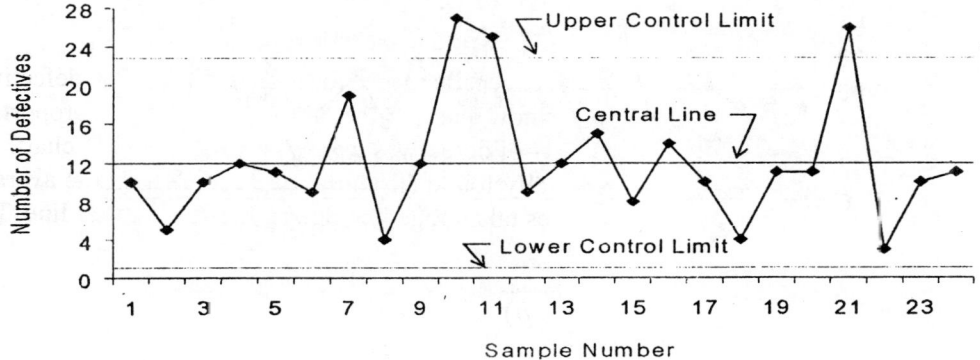

Evidently, sample numbers 10, 11 and 21 fall outside the upper control limit

(b) *p*-chart

$$CL = \bar{p} = 0.06$$

$$Control\ Limit = \bar{p} \pm 3\sqrt{\frac{\bar{p}(1-\bar{p})}{n}}$$

$$= 0.06 \pm 3\sqrt{\frac{0.06 \times 0.94}{200}}$$

$$= 0.009\ and\ 0.111$$

For showing the efectives proportion in various samples in the *p*-chart, we shall calculate their values in each of the samples. These are:

Sample No	Defectives	Sample No	Defectives	Sample No	Defectives
1	0.050	9	0.060	17	0.050
2	0.025	10	0.135	18	0.020
3	0.050	11	0.125	19	0.055
4	0.060	12	0.045	20	0.055
5	0.055	13	0.060	21	0.130
6	0.045	14	0.075	22	0.015
7	0.095	15	0.040	23	0.050
8	0.020	16	0.070	24	0.055

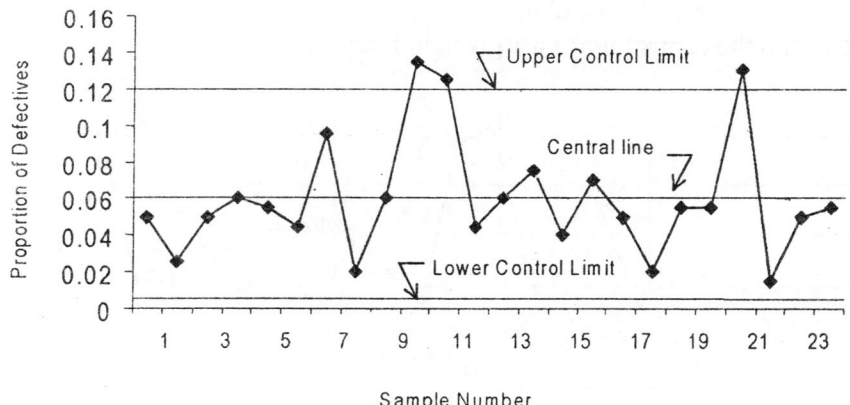

Here again, sample numbers 10, 11 and 21 are outside the upper control limit.

It may be mentioned here that when control chart is prepared on the basis of sample information, as in the above case, and some of the points lie beyond either of the control limits, then the control limits may be revised for use in the future. This is done by omitting those samples for which the values are outside the upper or the lower limits. In this example, the limits for the p-chart may be re-established by ignoring the sample numbers 10, 11 and 21. This gives:

$$\text{CL}: \quad \bar{p} = \frac{\text{No of defectives}}{\text{No of items examined}} = \frac{210}{21 \times 200} = 0.05$$

$$\text{Control Limits: } \bar{p} \pm 3\sqrt{\frac{\bar{p}(1-\bar{p})}{n}} = 0.05 \pm 3\sqrt{\frac{0.05 \times 0.95}{200}}$$

$$= \quad 0.004 \text{ and } 0.096$$

Now since all the sample proportions lie between the limits, these may be taken to the revised control limits for future.

(c)   **c-chart:** As already stated, a c-chart is prepared in situations where the focus is on the number of defects in different items. For construction of this chart, first the average number of defects, $\bar{c}$, is determined – either with the help of the past data, or from the samples of items examined. The control limits are determined by $\bar{c} \pm 3\sqrt{\bar{c}}$.

Example 6

The results of inspection of 40 pieces of an article give the mean number of defects to be 2.25. Find the 3-sigma control limits for the c-chart.

$$\text{Hence } \bar{c} = 2.25$$

$$\text{UCL}_c = \bar{c} + 3\sqrt{\bar{c}}$$
$$= 2.25 + 4.5 = 6.75$$

$$\text{LCL}_c = \bar{c} - 3\sqrt{\bar{c}}$$
$$= 2.25 - 4.5 = -2.5$$
$$= 0 \text{ (being negative)}$$

Example 7

The following table gives the inspection result of 25 similar glass tubes for the number of defects in them. Using these values, draw a c-chart.

Tube No.	1	2	3	4	5	6	7	8	9	10	11	12	13
Defects	2	1	2	6	8	2	4	9	3	4	5	3	3
Tube No	14	15	16	17	18	19	20	21	22	23	24	25	
Defects	7	4	5	2	4	3	7	2	4	5	3	2	

Total number of defects in all samples $=$ 100

Average number of defects $=$ $100/25 = 4$

$\therefore$ CL $= 4$

$$UCL_c = 4 + 3\sqrt{4}$$
$$= 4 + 6 = 10$$
$$LCL_c = 4 - 3\sqrt{4}$$
$$= 4 - 6 = -2 = 0$$

The c-chart is show in figure

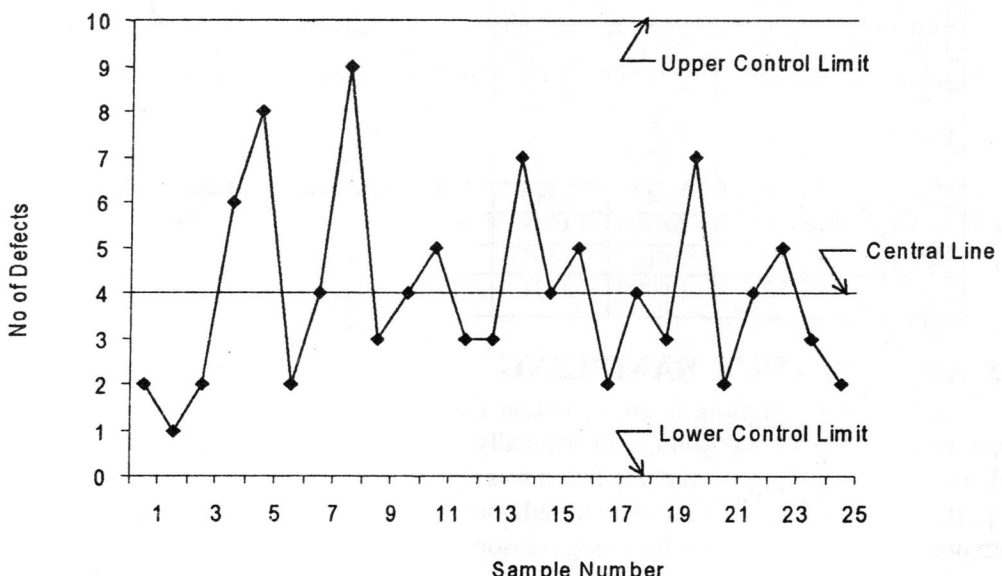

Since all the points lie between the control limits, the process is in control.

Table of Control Chart Constants

Sample Size = n	X-bar Chart Constants A_2	A_3	for sigma estimate d_2	R Chart Constants D_3	D_4	S Chart Constants B_3	B_4
2	1.880	2.659	1.128	—	3.267	—	3.267
3	1.023	1.954	1.693	—	2.574	—	2.568
4	0.729	1.628	2.059	—	2.282	—	2.266
5	0.577	1.427	2.326	—	2.114	—	2.089
6	0.483	1.287	2.534	—	2.004	0.030	1.970
7	0.419	1.182	2.704	0.076	1.924	0.118	1.882
8	0.373	1.099	2.847	0.136	1.864	0.185	1.815
9	0.337	1.032	2.970	0.184	1.816	0.239	1.761
10	0.308	0.975	3.078	0.223	1.777	0.284	1.716
11	0.285	0.927	3.173	0.256	1.744	0.321	1.679
12	0.266	0.886	3.258	0.283	1.717	0.354	1.646
13	0.249	0.850	3.336	0.307	1.693	0.382	1.618
14	0.235	0.817	3.407	0.328	1.672	0.406	1.594
15	0.223	0.789	3.472	0.347	1.653	0.428	1.572
16	0.212	0.763	3.532	0.363	1.637	0.448	1.552
17	0.203	0.739	3.588	0.378	1.622	0.466	1.534
18	0.194	0.718	3.640	0.391	1.608	0.482	1.518
19	0.187	0.698	3.689	0.403	1.597	0.497	1.503
20	0.180	0.680	3.735	0.415	1.585	0.510	1.490
21	0.173	0.663	3.778	0.425	1.575	0.523	1.477
22	0.167	0.647	3.819	0.434	1.566	0.534	1.466
23	0.162	0.633	3.858	0.443	1.557	0.545	1.455
24	0.157	0.619	3.895	0.451	1.548	0.555	1.445
25	0.153	0.606	3.931	0.459	1.541	0.565	1.435

3.5 ACCEPTANCE SAMPLING

Acceptance sampling is an important field of statistical quality control that was popularized by Dodge and Romig and originally applied by the U.S. military to the testing of bullets during World War II. If every bullet was tested in advance, no bullets would be left to ship. If, on the other hand, none were tested, malfunctions might occur in the field of battle, with potentially disastrous results. Dodge reasoned that a sample should be picked at random from the lot, and on the basis of information that was yielded by the sample, a decision should be made regarding the disposition of the lot. In general, the decision is either to accept or reject the lot. This process is called *Lot Acceptance Sampling* or just *Acceptance Sampling*.

An acceptance sampling plan is the overall scheme for either accepting or rejecting a lot based on information gained from samples, regarding the quality of the samples inspected.

Acceptance sampling is "the middle of the road" approach between no inspection and 100% inspection. There are two major classifications of acceptance plans: by *attributes* ("go, no-go") and by *variables*. The attribute case is the most common for acceptance sampling, and will be assumed for the rest of this section. A point to remember is that the main purpose of acceptance sampling is to decide whether or not the lot is likely to be acceptable, not to estimate the quality of the lot. Acceptance sampling is employed when one or several of the following hold:

- Testing is destructive
- The cost of 100% inspection is very high
- 100% inspection takes too long

It was pointed out by Harold Dodge in 1969 that Acceptance Quality Control is not the same as Acceptance Sampling. The latter depends on specific sampling plans, which when implemented indicate the conditions for acceptance or rejection of the immediate lot that is being inspected. The former may be implemented in the form of an Acceptance Control Chart. The control limits for the Acceptance Control Chart are computed using the specification limits and the standard deviation of what is being monitored .

A lot acceptance sampling plan (LASP) is a sampling scheme and a set of rules for making decisions. The decision, based on counting the number of defectives in a sample, can be to accept the lot, reject the lot, or even, for multiple or sequential sampling schemes, to take another sample and then repeat the decision process.

ACCEPTANCE SAMPLING PLANS

Acceptance sampling plan: a specific plan that clearly states the rules for sampling and the associated criteria for acceptance or otherwise. Acceptance sampling plans can be applied for inspection of (i) end items, (ii) components, (iii) raw materials, (iv) operations, (v) materials in process, (v) supplies in storage, (vi) maintenance operations, (vii) data or records and (viii) administrative procedures.

To ensure perfect quality, it is necessary to develop inspection and testing methods that re quick and effective so that all products are subjected to 100 percent inspection and testing. This means that every product shipped to customer is inspected and tested to determine whether it meets customer specifications. (i.e., design specification)/ But there are situations where it is either impossible or uneconomical to inspect and test each and every product, when destructive tests are called for or the quantity to be inspected or tested is quite large where 100 percent inspection or testing are uneconomical, impractical or impossible. In such situations, sampling inspection based on acceptance plans is the only sensible basis for inspecting and testing.

An acceptance plan is the overall scheme for either accepting or rejecting a lot based on information gained from samples, regarding the quality of the samples inspected. The acceptance plan identifies both the size and type of samples and the criteria to be used to used to either accept or reject this lot.

Acceptance Sampling is a form of inspection that is applied to lots or batches of items either before or after a process instead of during the process. The lot may represent incoming purchased items or raw materials, or semi-finished items (items that have completed certain manufacturing operations) or final products awaiting shipment to warehouses or customers. The purpose of acceptance sampling is to decide whether a lot satisfies predetermined quality standards or not. Based on the quality of the samples drawn from the lot, the lot is accepted or rejected. Rejected lots may be subjected to 100 percent inspection to segregate accepted or rejected. Rejected lots may be subjected to 100 percent inspection to segregate the defective items from the good ones. Acceptance sampling procedures are most useful when

(i) A large number of items must be processed in a short time.

(ii) Destructive testing is required and

(iii) Fatigue or boredom caused by inspecting large numbers of items leads to inspection errors.

Acceptance sampling procedures can be applied to inspection of both attribute and quality characteristics.

Sampling plans

A variety of sampling plans (acceptance plans) can be used. They are (i) Single sampling plan, (ii) double sampling plan and (iii) Sequential sampling plan.

a) Single sampling plan

In a single sampling plan, one random sample is drawn from each lot and every item in the sample is inspected or tested and classified as either "good" or "defective"/ If any sample contains more than a specified members of defectives 'C' (also referred to as acceptance number) that lot is rejected.

Exhibit : illustrates how single – sampling plans operate.

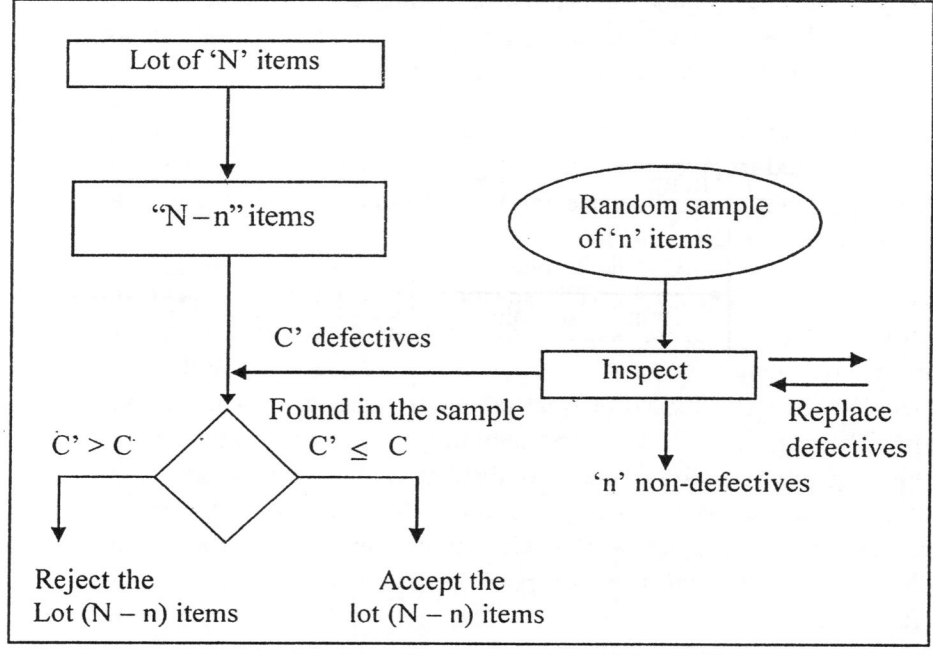

Single-sampling plans

b) Double Sampling Plan

A double sampling plan allows for the opportunity to take a second sample if the results of the initial sample are inconclusive. For example, if the number of defectives (C) is less than the acceptance number 'C', the lot is accepted, otherwise the lot is rejected and subjected to 100 percent inspection.

In order to reduce such 100 percent inspection, double sampling plans allow to draw a second sample from the rejected lot and subject the sample to inspection to take the decision to accept or reject the lot.

With double-sampling plan, two values are specified for the number of defective items (acceptance numbers), a lower level C_1 and the upper level C_2. If the number of defective items in the first sample is less than or equal to the lower values (i.e. C_1) the lot is accepted and the sampling is terminated. If the number of defectives exceeds the upper value (i.e. C_2) the lot is rejected. If the number of defective falls in between C_1 and C_2, a second sample is taken and the number of defectives in both samples is compared with C_2 and lot is accepted if the total number of defects in the two samples is less than or equal to C_2, otherwise the lot is rejected.

Exhibit   illustrates how a double-sampling plan for attributes operates

Double Sampling Plans

c) Sequential Sampling Plans (or Multisampling Plan)

In a sequential sampling plan, units (samples) are randomly selected from the lot and tested one by one. After each one has been tested, a reject, accept or continue, sampling decision is made. This process continues until the lot is accepted or rejected Exhibit 4.3 illustrates how such plans operate with attributes.

Exhibit : Sequential Sampling

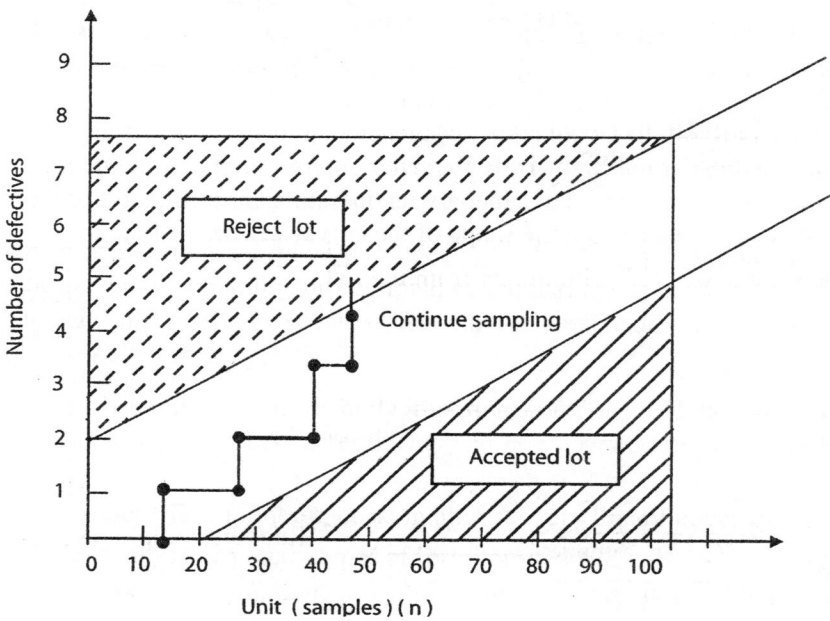

Plans

In the above exhibit, the first defective is the 15th unit, putting us in the continue sampling zone and we continue to sample units from the lot. The second defective is the 25th nit and we continue sampling the fourth defective is the 40th unit and this puts us in the reject zone, therefore the lot is rejected.

Choosing a sampling plan

The cost and time required for inspection often dictate the kind of sampling plan used. The two primary considerations are the number of samples needed and the total number of observations required. Single sampling plans involve only one sample, but the sample size is large relative to the total number of observations taken under double or multiple sampling plans.

Where the cost to obtain a sample is relatively high compared with the cost to analyse the observations, a single-sampling plan is recommended. Where item inspection costs are relatively high such as destructive testing it may be better to use double or multiple sampling because average number of items inspected per lot will be lower.

Single sampling plans for attributes

Two important concepts are needed to understand acceptance plans for attributes. They are:

(i)   Operating characteristic curves

(ii) Average outgoing quality curves..

Operating characteristic curve: An important feature of a sampling plan is how it discriminates between lots of high and low quality (i.e., good and bad lots). The ability of a sampling plan to discriminate is described by its operating characteristic (O.C) curve. The discriminating ability depends on the shape of the curve, which is a function of:

(i)   the sample size "n" with drawn from the lot.

(ii) The acceptance level or acceptance number of allowable defective units found in the sample

A typical O.C curve for a single sampling plan is shown in below Exhibit .

Exhibit   A typical operating characteristic curve

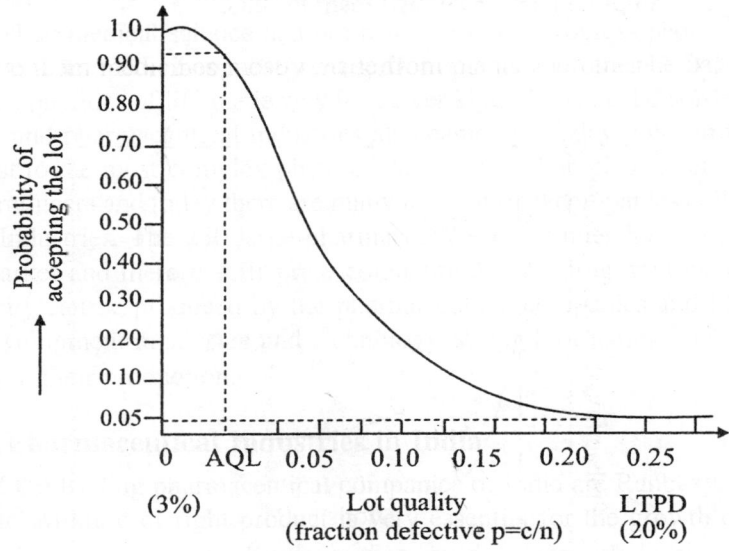

The O.C. curve shows the probability that use of the sampling plan will result in lots with various fraction defectives being accepted. For example, the graph shows that a lot with 3 percent defectives would have a probability of 0.90 (i.e. 90 percent) of being accepted

and a probability of 0.10 (i.e 10 percent) of being rejected. It may be noted from the shape of the curve that as lot quality decreases (i.e. fraction defective increases), the probability of acceptance of the lot decreases, although the relationship is not linear.

A sampling plan does not provide perfect discrimination between good and bad lots. There are four possible outcomes:

- Desirables (i) A good lot can be accepted

     (ii) A bad lot can be rejected.

- Undesirable (i) a good lot may be rejected

     (ii) A bad lot may be accepted.

It can be seen from the graph that a lot having more than 20 percent defectives (a bad lot) still has some probability of acceptance (say 5%) whereas a lot with a high quality (low percent defective, say 3%) has some chance getting rejected (say probability of 0.1 or 10%)

The degree to which a sampling plan discriminates between good and bad lots is a function of the steepness of the graph's O.C. curve, the steeper the curve, the more discriminating the sampling plan. Exhibit illustrates this.

Exhibit :   OC Curve for discriminating between good and bad lots

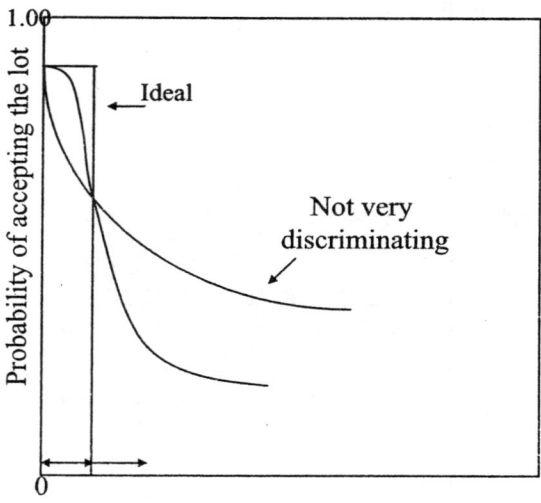

"Good" "Bad"   Lot quality (fraction defective)

The curve for an ideal plan (i.e ideal O.C. curve) can perfectly discriminate between good and bad lots. To achieve this degree of discrimination, 100 percent inspection of each lot is necessary. Because of the cost and time needed for 100 percent inspection, it is often rule out, leaving acceptance sampling as the only viable alternative.

For these reasons, buyers (consumers) are generally willing to accept lot that contain small percentage of defective items as "good" lots especially if the cost related to a few defective is low. Of ten this percentage is between 1 and 2 percent defective. This figure (fraction defective) is known as acceptance quality level (AQL) or acceptable quality level.

Because of the inability of random sampling to clearly identify lots that contain more than specified percentage of defectives, consumers recognize that some lots that actually contain more defectives will be accepted based on the sample evidence. However, there is usually an upper limit on the percentage of defectives that a customer is willing to tolerate in accepted lots. This is known as lot tolerance percent defective (LTPD). Thus, consumers want lot quality to be equal to or better than AL and are willing to live with some lots the LTPD will be accepted is known s consumer's risk. (â) or the probability of making a type II error. The probability that a lot containing acceptable quality level (AQL) will be rejected is known as the producer's risk (á) or the probability of making a type I error. Many sampling plans are designed to have a producer's risk of 5 percent and a consumer's risk of 10 percent. although other combinations are also used. It is possible by trial and error to design a plan that will provide selected values for á and â given the AQL and the LTPD. Below Exhibit 6 illustrates an O.C, curve with the AQL, LTPD, producer's risk and consumer's risk.

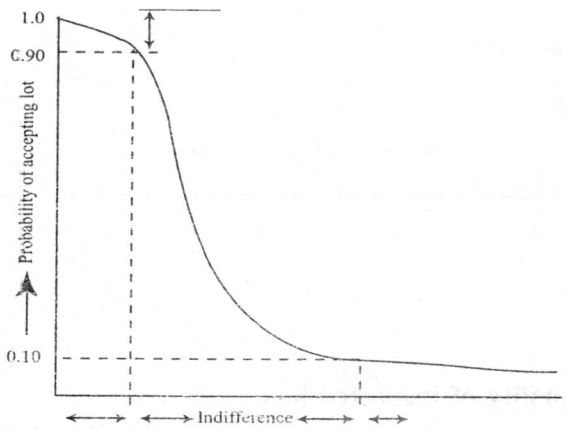

Lot quality (percent defective)

Exhibit   Typical O.C.Curve

The type I and type II errors can be avoided or reduced by the following:

(i)   Sample must be taken in ways that allow them to be truly random, thus improving the likelihood that sample will be representative of lots,

(ii)   By increasing the sample size (n)

Exhibit shows the effect of sample size on the o.c. curve

Probability of Accepting Lots (percent)

Exhibit: OC curves for different sample sizes and acceptance numbers (i.e., n and c)

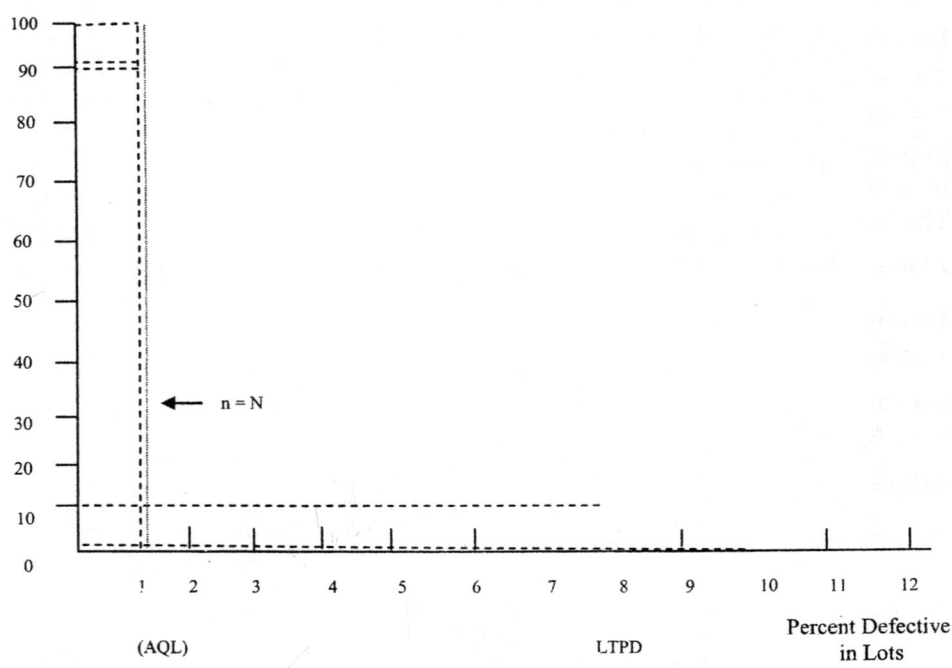

Average outgoing quality of inspected lots

An interesting feature of acceptance sampling is that the level of inspection automatically adjusts to the quality of lots being inspected; assuming rejected lots are subjected to 100 percent inspection. The O.C. curve reveals that the greater the percentage of defectives in a lot, the less likely the lot is to be accepted. Good lots have a high probability and bad lots have a low probability of being accepted. If the lots inspected are mostly good, few will end up going through 100 percent inspection. The poorer the quality of the lots, the greater the number of lots that will come under close scrutiny. This tends to improve overall quality of lots by weeding out defectives. In this way, the level of inspection is affected by lot quality.

If all lots have some given fraction defective 'p' the average outgoing quality (AOQ) of the lots can be computed using the following formula, assuming defectives are replaced with good items.

$$AOQ= P_{ac} \times p\left(\frac{N-n}{N}\right)$$

Where P_{ac} =Probability of accepting the lot

P= Fraction defective

N= Lot size

N= Sample size

In practice, the last term is often omitted since it is usually close to 1.0 and therefore has little effect on the resulting values.

The formula then becomes

$$AOQ= P_{ac} \times p$$

Example of construction of AOQ curve

N=500, n=10,C=1

Let value of p vary from 0.05 to 0.40 in steps of 0.05. The probabilities of acceptance P_{ac} from Appendix Table D is given below

$$AOQ= P_{ac} \times p$$

P	P_{ac}	AOQ
0.05	0.9137	0.046
0.10	0.7361	0.074
0.15	0.5443	0.082
0.20	0.3758	0.075
0.25	0.2440	0.061
0.30	0.1493	0.045
0.35	0.0860	0.030
0.40	0.0464	0.019

Exhibit   Construction of AOQ curve

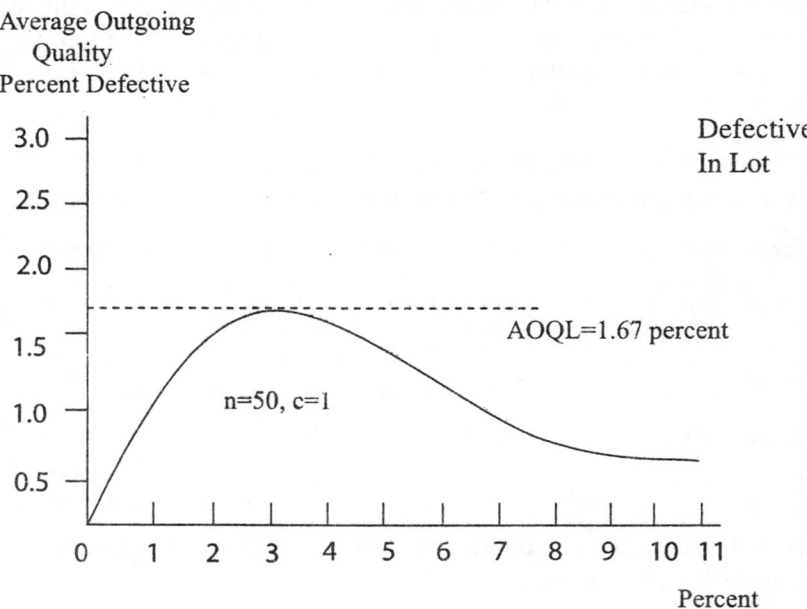

Average Outgoing
   Quality
Percent Defective

The AOQ curve illustrates the point that if lots very good or very bad, the average outgoing quality will be high. The maximum point on the curve becomes apparent in the process of calculating values for the curve.

The several implications of the graph are:

1.   Manager can determine the worst possible outgoing quality.

2.   the manager can determine the amount of inspection that will be needed by obtaining an estimate of the incoming quality. The manager can use this information to establish the relationship between inspection cost and incoming fraction defective, thereby underscoring the benefits by implementing the process improvements to reduce the incoming fraction defective rather than trying to weed out bad items through inspection.

3.6 DEMING'S CONTRIBUTION TO QUALITY

Deming's principles of quality improvement.

1)   Establish a goal of continuous innovation and improvement.

2) Adopt a philosophy that does not tolerate mistakes, delays, or defects.

3) Cease dependence upon mass inspection; require statistical evidence of quality.

4) End the practice of awarding business on the basis of price.

5) Search continuously to uncover problems (e.g., using statistical methods).

6) Institute modern methods of training on the job.

7) Refocus supervisors' attention from quantity to quality that will improve productivity.

8) Drive out fear, so that everyone feels secure and encouraged to seek improvement.

9) Break down departmental barriers and those with suppliers and customers.

10) Eliminate posters and slogans that don't actually help people solve problems.

11) Eliminate work standards that prescribe numerical quotas.

12) Remove barriers that stand between worker and their right to pride in workmanship.

13) Institute a vigorous retraining program to keep up with changes.

14) Create a top management structure that will push every day for the above 13 points.

The main objective of quality control is the prevention of defects in manufacturing. So that the units produced meet product quality specifications right at the first time they are manufactured and not have to be reworked or rejected. That is, it aims at producing products, which are dependable, economical and satisfactory.

To achieve the above said objective quality management should be taken as a continuous improvement programme. The concept of Deming's circle, enunciated by Dr.W.Edwards Deming explains the improvement process as shown in the following Figure

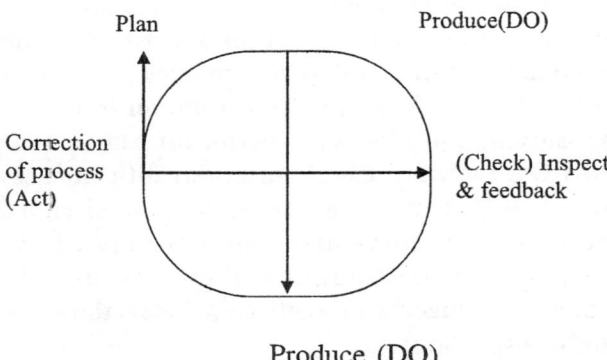

Produce (DO)

Fig : Deming's Circle – PDCA cycle.

The above figure can be elaborated in six stages. They are:

1) Set quality standards.

2) Plan methods, technology, materials tooling and personnel to achieve the specified quality.

3) Manufacture right the first time.

4) Inspect and report any quality short comings.

5) Carryout corrections in process, control, tooling, etc.

6) Re-plan for long term quality control.

An organisation that is committed to quality must examine quality at three levels, namely, i) the organizational level, ii) the process level and iii) the performer or job or task-des level.

SUMMARY:

Work study is a generic term for those techniques, particularly method study and work measurement, which are used in the examination of human work in all its contents, and which lead systematically to the investigation of all the factors which affect the efficiency and economy of the situation being reviewed, in order to effect improvement. Statistical quality control measures the variation in during the process which can be controlled after rectifying causes for variation. The control charts are available for variables and attributes. The quality control for the incoming and finished goods is done with Acceptance sampling methods. Organizations are growing increasingly conscious of competitive potential of quality, which has now become a new competitive weapon. Deming, Juran and Crosby who are known as quality gurus advocated quality control and quality management as a new philosophy and the decade of 1980 was a decade of quality revolution in the U.S The purpose of quality control is to assure that processes are performing in an acceptable manner. Some of the widely used QC tools are Check sheet, Stratification, Pareto diagram, Ishikawa diagram, histogram, Scatter diagram and Control chart. This chapter presents lot-by-lot acceptance sampling plans for attributes, Key topics include the design and operation of single sampling plans, the use of the operating characteristic curve, and the concepts of rectifying inspection, average outgoing quality and average total inspection.

REVIEW QUESTIONS:

i).   Define 'work study' and describe the steps involved in the procedure to carry out work study in an organisation..

ii).   State the applications of work study. Describe the procedure of work study.

iii). Define work study, Method Study and work Measurement. Explain the interrelationship between them.

iv).   Define Quality, Quality Control?

v).   Explain the Edwards Deming's 14 points of improving quality?

vi).   Describe Deming's Circle (PDCA Cycle) in brief?

vii). What is OC curve? Discuss the acceptance sampling methods

viii). What do you mean the term SQC? What are its benefits to the organisation?

ix).   What is control chart? What are the types of control charts?

x).   From the following data construct control charts for Mean and Range and comment.

Sample observations	Sample observations				
tions	1	2	3	4	5
1	1.01	1.02	1.02	0.98	1.04
2	0.97	0.99	1.01	0.95	0.97
3	1.04	1.02	1.01	1.00	1.00
4	1.03	1.01	0.97	0.98	0.99
5	1.00	1.02	0.98	1.01	1.01
6	1.00	1.01	0.99	0.99	0.95
7	0.99	1.02	1.03	1.01	0.97
8	0.96	0.95	1.02	1.03	1.01
9	0.93	0.98	0.99	1.04	1.04
10	1.05	1.05	0.97	1.02	0.99

xi)   Circular brass discs were inspected before reaching the assembly line. Nominal thickness (specified) is 11mm with ± 0.2 mm tolerance. Hourly inspections by samples gave the results as shown below

Sample Number	Measurement (from) per sample in			
	1	2	3	4
1	8.7	10.5	9.7	9.5
2	10.0	8.3	10.1	10.1
3	11.3	9.2	11.2	9.8
4	11.3	9.5	9.4	9.3
5	10.1	10.7	8.8	8.7
6	9.2	9.5	11.1	10.6
7	9.0	10.2	11.5	9.0
8	9.9	10.0	10.2	10.2
9	8.2	10.9	10.5	11.6
10	8.9	9.9	10.5	9.0
11	10.3	11.0	10.6	8.6
12	8.6	11.5	9.6	8.9
13	10.0	9.2	9.8	10.5
14	7.5	11.3	10.3	11.0
15	10.5	8.4	8.4	10.0
16	11.5	9.2	10.1	10.8
17	12.4	11.5	11.4	8.9
18	9.7	10.2	9.8	9.3

The assembly persons complained that the thickness was out of control. Draw Mean and range charts and make your comments on the process. Use $A_2 = 0.73$, $D_3 = 0$ and $D_4 = 2.28$.

xii) The following data relate to the day- by – day output of castings for 10 days. Construct appropriate control chart and comment.

Day	1	2	3	4	5	6	7	8	9	10
No. of castings produced	150	154	145	154	150	145	145	154	152	152
No. of defective castings	2	4	2	4	3	4	2	2	1	4

xiii)   Ten assemblies were inspected and the defects per assembly are shown below. Determine the control limits for the defects per assembly.

Sample Number	1	2	3	4	5	6	7	8	9	10
Defects	6	4	1	4	8	0	2	0	4	3

xiv). Twenty samples of cloth each of equal length and width were examined in order to launch a quality control program. The number of defects observed per sample are as shown below: With the help of a suitable control chart discuss whether the process is in control?

Sample Number	Number of defectives	Sample Number	Number of defectives
1	1	11	2
2	4	12	5
3	4	13	9
4	1	14	8
5	6	15	4
6	3	16	2
7	5	17	7
8	10	18	2
9	7	19	6
10	3	20	4

xv). The probabilities of acceptance of the lots(of uniform size) under an acceptance sampling plan are given as follows. Draw the OPERATING CHARESTERISTIC Curve and mark the following: i) AQL at 5% Producers' Risk. ii) LTPD at 5% Consumers' Risk. And indicate their respective values.

Actual Percent defectives in the submitted lots	Probability of Acceptance
2.4	0.731
2.8	0.650
3.2	0.570
3.6	0.494
4.0	0.424
5.0	0.278
6.0	0.174
7.0	0.106
8.0	0.062
10.0	0.020
12.0	0.006

Chapter 4

ORGANIZATION OF DISTRIBUTION AND MARKETING

4.1 INTRODUCTION

Widely used definition of marketing is- "Marketing is a social and managerial process by which individuals and groups obtain what they need and want through creating and exchanging products and value with others." (Kotler & Armstrong 1987)

The mission of marketing is satisfying **customer needs.** That takes place in a social context. In developed societies marketing is needed in order to satisfy the needs of society's members. Industry is the tool of society to produce products for the satisfaction of needs.

There are broad and narrow definitions of marketing. Different types of approaches to marketing are needed when analyzing the possibilities to improve marketing. Marketing has a **connective function in society**. It connects supply and demand or production and consumption. At micro-level, marketing builds and maintains the relationship between producer and consumer. At business unit level, marketing can have **an integrative function**. It integrates all the functions and parts of a company to serve the markets. The narrowest definition is to see marketing as **a function of a business enterprise** between production and markets taking care that products move smoothly from production to customers.

4.2 THE SOCIETAL FUNCTION OF MARKETING

In modern society production and consumption are apart from each other. Marketing connects them. From the societal point of view, marketing is a philosophy which shows how to create effective production systems and consequently prosperity.

Business is a subsystem of society, which has both a social and an economic role. Thus, a company must operate in a way that will make possible the production of benefits for society and, at the same time, produce profits for the company itself. The role of marketing in society means also responsibilities. In addition to economic and social responsibility, ecological responsibility is nowadays emphasized. According to some definitions, environmental responsibility is part of social responsibility. Improvement of marketing is related to the changing emphases of economic, social and environmental responsibility.

The traditional and integrating functions of marketing

Traditionally, marketing has been seen as a link between production and customer. The situation could be captured better by using the term selling. Selling is associated to the so- called "Production and Sales Eras of Marketing". Slogans: "Make what you can make" and "Get rid of what you have made" describe the traditional view of marketing/selling.

The following figure shows the role of traditionally oriented marketing in (traditionally oriented) management.

Marketing was born out of a need to take better into consideration the demand factors in production planning. The function of marketing is to channel information of consumer needs to the production and satisfaction of needs to consumers. The basic power of marketing is the aspiration to produce and sell only that kind of products which have demand. Marketing integrates the whole company to serve this demand. Marketing aims at effective production systems, where information is transmitted effectively between production and consumption.

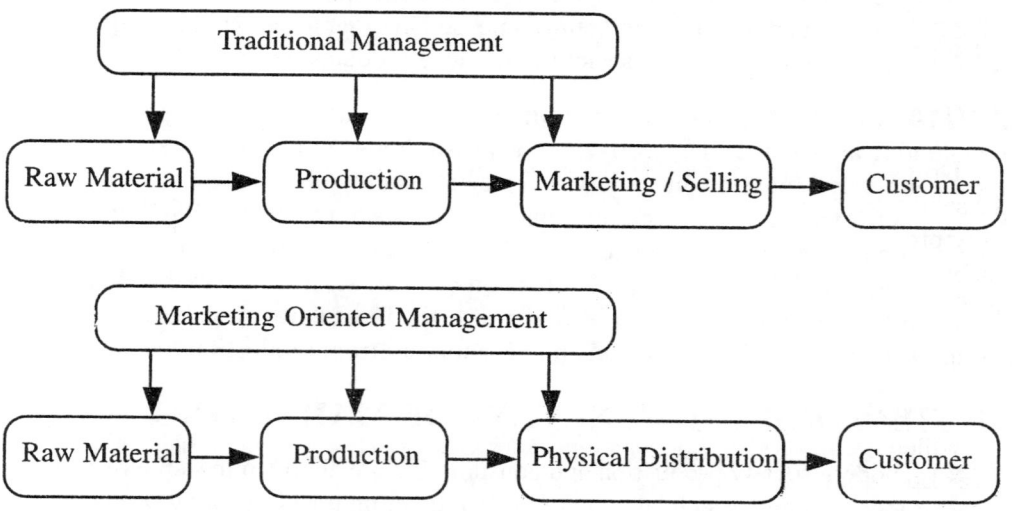

There are eight universal functions performed in marketing:

1. Buying: (Raw material to produce goods and services and to purchase finished goods or services as retailer or wholesaler to sell them again for final customers and consumers). It is a function that ensures that product offerings are available in sufficient quantities to meet customer demands.

2. Selling: The function to be performed to sell the products/services/idea to satisfy customer needs or wants by using advertising, personal selling and sales promotion to match goods and services to customer needs.

3. Transporting: Function related to create the availability of product or services. It is used for moving products from their points of production to location convenient for purchases

4. Storing: Warehouses are used to store the products for further distribution.

5. Standardizing and grading: To provide more quality products and services without variation in the quality. Ensuring that product offerings meet established and grading quality and quantity control standards of size, weight, and other product variables.

6. Financing: Providing the financial resources to carry out different promotion of product and providing credit for channel members (wholesaler's retailers) or consumers.

7. Risk taking: Marketer takes a risk specifically when any new product is introduced in a market because there are equal chances of success and failure. Dealing with uncertainty about consumer purchases resulting from creation and marketing of goods and services that consumers may purchase in the future.

4.3 PHARMACEUTICAL MARKETING

Drugs and pharmaceuticals are required by rich and poor alike for removing diseases and disabilities. Hence drugs should be available at a cheaper rate and accessible to everyone. Simply producing quality medicines is not sufficient. Their distribution and making them available when required is also very important. Hence pharmaceutical marketing is a potential force that commands high significance for the country as a whole.

The following are important factors in pharmaceutical marketing:

1. Drugs and pharmaceuticals are related to nation health care policy. An increase in the efficiency of pharmaceutical marketing results in a lower cost of distribution. Lower prices to patients means a real increase in the national income

2. Due to efficient pharmaceutical marketing activity, a decrease in the prices of drugs and pharmaceuticals will make even a poor man to afford for purchase of medicines.

3. Pharmaceutical marketing makes available life saving drugs and medicines which enhance the life span of people thereby rising the standard of living of people

4. In our country, a total of 75,000 crores of drugs and pharmaceuticals are produced. This activity gives job opportunities and livelihood to several thousand people

The following are the important objectives of pharmaceutical marketing:

- To provide guiding policies for marketing of drugs and pharmaceuticals
- To study the problems associated with the marketing of drugs and pharmaceuticals and to suggest solutions
- To enable successful distribution of drugs, pharmaceuticals and medicinal products
- To analyze the shortcomings in the existing pattern of pharmaceutical marketing

The following table gives the major differences between general (consumer) marketin and pharmaceutical marketing

GENERAL MARKETING	PHARMACEUTICAL MARKETING
Consumer Is The Ultimate Decision Maker	The doctor or physician is the decision maker
No control of government on quality of items	The quality of medicines is stringently controlled by the government.
Audio visual media is used for advertising the products	Advertising of drugs and medicines is strictly prohibited by law.
General/marketing sales personnel do not require special and qualified people	It is usually done by personal approach
No shelf-life and no expiry date for general goods	Only science and pharmacy graduates are utilized as representatives. Hence specialized people are required for pharmaceutical marketing
General /marketing sales personnel do not require special and qualified people	Shelf-life and expiry date is fixed and legal control is there over the issue
Obsolescence is very fast (change in the trend and fashions)	No such obsolescence
Prescription is not required for purchasing consumer goods	A prescription from a qualified physician is mandatory for purchase of medicines Consumer does not have a choice
Consumer has several options and choices Licenses are not mandatory except for sales license	Licenses are required for distribution and selling of drugs

Table: General Marketing Vs Pharmaceutical Marketing

The following diagram gives the marketing activities in pharmaceutical industry.

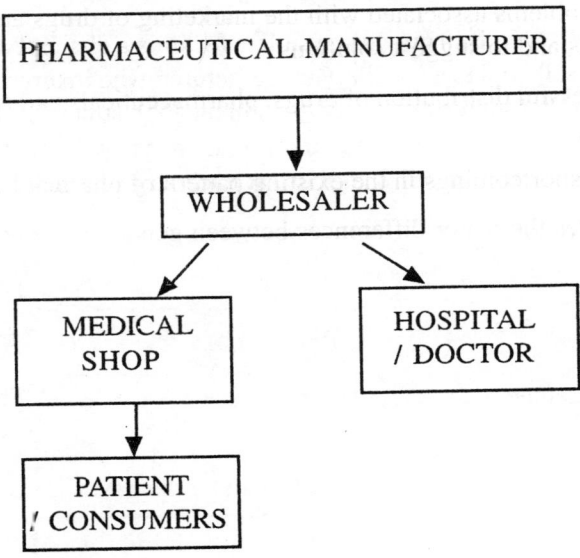

Figure : Pharmaceutical marketing

4.4 MARKETING MIX

Marketing mix consist of 4Ps which are the ideas to consider when marketing a product. They form the basis of the marketing mix. Getting this mix right is critical in order to successfully market a product. The 4Ps are:

1. Product
2. Price
3. Promotion
4. Place

If market research is carried out effectively, a company can plan a promotion for the right product, at the right price, and to get it to their chosen market, in the right place.

Product

A product can be either a good or a service that is sold either to a commercial customer or an end consumer. A customer buys a product, and a consumer uses it. Sometimes these are one and the same, as an industrial firm can also be a customer and a consumer. For example, British Airways might buy aero planes from British Aerospace, so it is a customer.

It won't sell on the planes to another buyer, as BA needs the planes to provide its service, so it is also a consumer. Sometimes a wide product range covers both (Mercedes produce lorries for haulage companies, and cars for domestic use).

More commonly, there will be a number of sellers forming a chain of distribution. For example, a gold mine may sell gold to a jewellery manufacturer, who in turn will sell on rings to wholesalers and retailers, before we get to buy them in the high street. Each is a customer, but only the final user is the end consumer. A marketing manager will identify who his/her target market is, what they want, and sell it to them at each stage in the chain.

The product is a combination of:

- Quality
- Design
- Name
- Warranty and guarantee
- Packaging
- Labeling
- Exclusive features

Customer service is important at this stage. Ongoing customer service, especially for complex and expensive products, is crucial for maintaining a strong customer relationship

The packaging is also important. It helps to promote the product and encourage first-time buyers to purchase it

Price

No matter how good the product is, it is unlikely to succeed unless the price is right. This does not just mean being cheaper than competitors. Most people associate a higher price with quality, so you would expect to pay more for a Rolls Royce than for a Lada. On the other hand, is one cola worth more than another, and if so, how much?

As a rule, a producer of luxury or medical products will use skim pricing or premium pricing initially, in order to maximize its profits. This is useful, as it helps them to recover expensive research and development costs quickly.

For fast moving consumable goods (FMCG's) like colas, penetration pricing is usually used. The firm will want a large share of the market, so will settle for a small profit on each item. In the long term, they hope that the turnover, and therefore their profits, will be high. The simplest method of all is cost-plus pricing , where a firm adds a profit mark-up to the unit cost.

If the price is too high, it could lead to lost sales (unless superior customer service is offered). If price is too low, it could give the impression of a 'cheap and nasty' product.

4 methods of calculating price:

1. Cost plus margin- calculating total cost of production plus adding a percentage (margin) for profit

2. Market price- pricing according to the interaction between quantities the customers is willing to purchase and the quantity that producers are willing to supply. Shortage of product= high price, surplus of product = low price

3. Competitors price- price that's either below, equal to or above competitors

4. Discount price- reducing the price to stimulate demand

Promotion

The main aims of promotion are to persuade, inform and make people more aware of a brand, as well as improving sales figures. Advertising is the most widely used form of promotion, and can be through the media of TV, radio, journals, cinema or outdoors (billboards, posters). The specific sections of society (market segments) being targeted will affect the types of media chosen, as will the cost. If you were a toy manufacturer, you might want an advertising spot during children's TV. If you ran a local restaurant, you might choose a local paper or radio.

A small or local business would not usually advertise on TV, because it is very expensive. Sales promotion is designed to encourage new and repeat sales. Loyalty cards, free gifts, competitions and voucher schemes are the most popular. Companies use sponsorship and public relations to improve their image, notably through financing sports, the arts and public information services.

A promotion strategy details the methods that a business uses to inform, persuade and remind customers about its products. The 4 main forms of promotion are:

1. Personal Selling- sales assistant outlines the features of the good or service to the customer.

2. Sales promotion- activities and materials used to attract interest and support for the good or service. E.g. free samples, coupons with cash refunds, loyalty programs (e.g. Fly bys)

3. Publicity- the business sets up a free news story about the product. The aim is to enhance the image of the product and the business

4. Advertising- print or electronic mass media used to communicate a message about the product.

The internet, use of E-commerce, online chat rooms, etc have also proven to be successful in the promotion of products

Place

Distribution channels are the key to this area. A firm has to find the most cost-effective way to get the product to the consumer. Direct marketing through catalogues, via a TV shopping channel and through the Internet have become popular, because the consumer can shop from home.

For the firm, they can cut out the middleman in the process, and can therefore make more profit. Going through wholesalers and high-street retailers, however, is the most popular form of distribution, as that is still where most people shop.

Where is the product going to be distributed? The business owner needs to decide how to transport and store the finished products. They also must decide on how many intermediaries (middle agents) to involve in the distribution of the product (example: wholesalers and retailers). Distribution can be exclusive or as wide as possible.

A firm will gather information about the marketplace (e.g. whether house prices are rising or falling), and then research consumers' needs. From this, it will identify who its market is, and then put together a marketing plan based on the findings. The marketing mix will be central to this, and finding the right balance in each of the 4Ps is very important. The firm can then reviews and adapt their plan when they need to. You should remember the following points:

- Although marketing is consumer-orientated, the main aim is still to be profitable.

- A good marketing manager will try to differentiate their product (i.e. make their product stand out against similar competitive brands).

- Whatever pricing decision is made, the most important factor is to breakeven.

- Making it as easy as possible for the customer to buy the product will help sales to increase.

4.5 MARKETING STATEGIES AND PRODUCT LIFE CYCLE

The marketing strategies are the actions that are undertaken to achieve the marketing objectives through the marketing mix.

The product life cycle plays and important role in marketing. Depending on which stage the product is at in its lifecycle will determine which element of the 4P's will have the most emphasis. If the product is just being introduced, a different marketing strategy will be required compared to if it was in its decline stage.

Companies normally reformulate their marketing strategies several times during a product's life. Changing economic conditions, launching a new product by the competitors, buyers' interest and other factors push a company to launch a new product in the market. Therefore, a company must plan strategies appropriate for each stages of its life cycle. We will focus on different stages of product's life cycle and strategies.

Product Life-Cycle

Product life cycle is the course of a product's sales and profits over its lifetime. It involves five distinct stages: Product Development, Introduction, Growth, Maturity, Decline.

People who believe products have a life cycle are making four claims:

1. Products have a limited life.

2. Product sales pass through distinct stages, each posing different challenges, opportunities, and problems to the seller.

3. Profits rise and fall at different stages of the product life cycle.

4. Products require different marketing, financial, manufacturing, purchasing, and human resource strategies in each stage of their life cycle.

Most products are seen as having a bell-shaped life cycle of product.

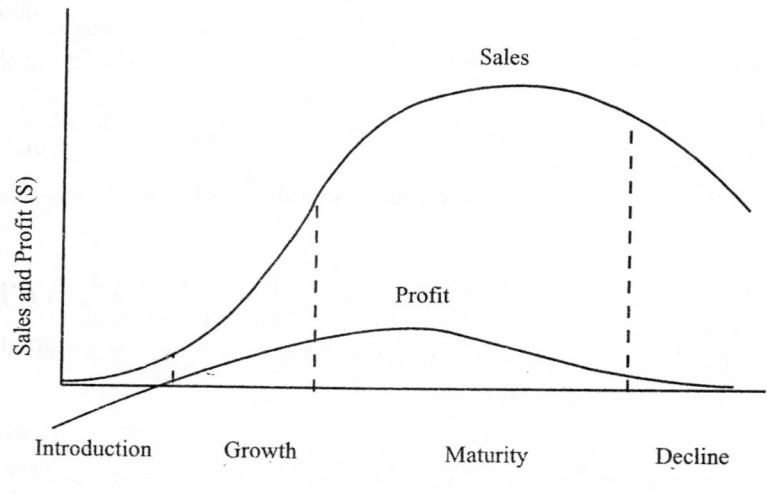

As a product moves from introduction, to growth, to maturity, and finally to decline, companies need to make adjustments in response to the changed circumstances.

1. **Introduction:** A period of slow sales growth as the product is introduced n the market. Profit are nonexistent I this stage because of the heavy expenses incurred with product introduction.

2. **Growth:** A period of rapid market acceptance and substantial profit improvement.

3. **Maturity:** A period of slowdown in sales growth because the product has achieved acceptance by most potential buyers. Profits stabilize or decline because of increased competition.]

4. **Decline:** The period when sales show a downward drift and profits erode.

MARKETING STRATEGIES IN VARIOUS STAGES OF PLC.

Introduction Stage

In this stage promotional expenditure remains higher because the company wants to a) inform the potential consumers, b) initiate pilot project (trial of product) and c) secure distribution n retail outlets.

Marketers can take one of the four strategies considering price and promotion.

1. *Rapid Skimming:* Launching a new product at a high price and high promotion level. This strategy makes sense when a large part of the potential consumers are unaware about the product.

2. *Slow Skimming:* Launching a new product at a high price and low promotion. This strategy makes sense when the market is limited in size. Most of the market is aware of the product, willing to pay even at a high price and potential competition is not imminent.

3. *Rapid Penetration:* Launching the product at a low price and spending heavily on promotion. This strategy makes sense when the market is large, the market is unaware of the product, most buyers are price sensitive, competition is strong, unit manufacturing cost falls in company's scale of production and company gains the benefit of experience.

4. *Slow Penetration:* Launching a new product at a low price and low promotional expenses. This strategy makes sense when the market is large and highly aware of the product, market is price sensitive and there is a chance of potential competitors.

Growth Stage:

As in the growth stage sales climb up and even at a higher rate considering to promotional expenses and new competitor emerged in this stage therefore, a company needs to make some careful strategies. Companies have several options:

1. It can improve the quality of the product, can add new product features or style.

2. It can add new models with different sizes, flavors, colors and so forth.

3. It can enter in to a new market segment.

4. It can enter in a new distribution channel or can increase the coverage of distribution.

5. Advertising message should focus on 'Product Preference Advertising' rather than 'Product Awareness Advertising'.

6. It may lower the price of the product in order to attract the next layer of the consumer group.

Maturity Stage:

The maturity stage can be divided into three parts: growth, stable and decaying maturity. However, the company can adopt 3 strategies in this stage.

1. *Market Modification:* The company can try to increase its over all sales volume either by increasing "number of brand users" or by increasing "usage rate per user". The company can try to expand the brand users by **converting non-users, entering new market segments, and winning competitors' customers.**

2. *Product Modification:* Products can be modified in three ways **quality improvement, feature improvement** and **style improvement.**

3. *Marketing Mix Modification:* Modifying marketing mix elements and sub-elements, a company can also take strategies at this stage. It includes **Prices, Distribution, Adverting, Sales Promotion, Personal Selling,** and **Services.**

Declining Stage:

Every product soon or later faces this stage. A company a can take several steps:

1. *Increase the firm's investment.*

2. *Maintaining the firm's investment.*

3. *Decreasing the firm's investment level selectively.*

4. *Harvesting – Picking-up the firm's investment to recover cash quickly.*

5. *Divesting – Disposing of its assets.*

Product Life Cycle: Characteristics, Marketing Objectives and Strategies

Characteristics	Introduction	Growth	Maturity	Decline
Sales	Low Sales	Rapidly Rising Sales	Peak Sales	Declining Sales
Costs	High Cost Per Customer	Avg. Cost Per Customer	Low Cost Per Customer	Low Cost Per Customer
Profits	Negative	Rising Profits	High Profits	Declining Profits
Customers	Innovators	Early Adopters	Middle Majority	Laggards
Competitors	Few	Growing Numbers	Stable Numbers	Decline Numbers
Marketing Objectives	**Create Product Awareness And Trial**	**Maximize Market Share**	**Maximize Profit While Defending Market Share**	**Reduce Expenditure**

Strategies

Product	Offer A Basic Product	Offer Product Extensions, Service And Warranty	Diversify Brands and items	Phase Out Weak Models
Price	Charge cost-plus Pricing Strategy	Penetration Pricing Strategy	Competition Based Strategy	Discount/Sales Promotion/Price Cut Strategy
Distribution	Build Selective Distribution	Build Intensive Distribution	Build More Intensive Distribution	Selective And Phase Out Unprofitable Outlets
Advertising	Build Product Awareness Among Early Adopters And Dealers	Build Awareness And Interest In The Mass-Market	Stress Brand Differences And Benefits	Maintain Relationship With The Loyal Groups
Sales Promotion	Heavy Sales Promotion	Reduce Promotional Expenditure	Increase To Encourage Brand Switching	Reduce To Minimal Level

4.6 ORGANISATION OF DISTRIBUTION

Marketing channels (Distribution channels) move goods and services for producers to consumers. It overcomes the major time, place and possession gaps the separate good and services from those who would use them. Manufacturers, wholesalers, and retailers as well other channels members exist in channel arrangements to perform one or more of the following generic functions:

1. Information gathering and distributing marketing research and intelligence information about actors and forces in the marketing environment needed for planning and aiding exchange.

2. Promotion: Developing and spreading persuasive communications about an offer.

3. Contact: Finding and communicating with prospective buyers.

4. Matching: Shaping and fitting the offer to the buyers needs including activities such as manufacturing, grading, assembling and packaging

5. Negotiation: Reaching an agreement on price and other terms of the offer so that ownership or possession can be transferred.

6. Others help to fulfill the completed transactions.

7. Physical distribution: Transporting and storing goods.

8. Financing: Acquiring and using funds to cover the costs of the channel work

9. Risk taking: assuming the risks of carrying out the channel work

10. Carrying of inventory, demand generation or selling, after sales services.

In getting its goods to end users, a manufacturer must either assume all these functions or shift some or all of them to channel intermediaries.

Channels

A number of alternate 'channels' of distribution may be available:

- Selling direct, such as with an outbound sales force or via mail order, Internet and telephone sales

- Agent, who typically sells direct on behalf of the producer

- Distributor (also called wholesaler), who sells to retailers

- Retailer (also called dealer or reseller), who sells to end customers

- Advertisement typically used for consumption goods

Distribution channels may not be restricted to physical products alone. They may be just as important for moving a service from producer to consumer in certain sectors, since both direct and indirect channels may be used. Hotels, for example, may sell their services (typically rooms) directly or through travel agents, tour operators, airlines, tourist boards, centralized reservation systems, etc.

There have also been some innovations in the distribution of services. For example, there has been an increase in <u>franchising</u> and in rental services - the latter offering anything from televisions through tools. There has also been some evidence of service integration, with services linking together, particularly in the travel and tourism sectors. For example, links now exist between airlines, hotels and car rental services. In addition, there has been a significant increase in retail outlets for the service sector. Outlets such as estate agencies and building society offices are crowding out traditional grocers from major shopping areas.

Channels can be classifies as:

1. Manufacturer → Consumer - Direct Marketing

2. Manufacturer → Retailer → Consumer – one stage

3. Manufacturer → Wholesaler → Retailer → Consumer – two stage

4. Manufacturer → Distributor → Wholesaler → Retailer → Consumer – three stage

1. Producer and consumer or direct sale (zero stage marketing)

Direct selling of goods and services by the manufacturer to the consumer. The producers establish connection with the consumers' directly through door to door salesmen, direct mail or by its own retail outlets.

Direct selling is gaining ground now a days because of exorbitant distribution costs through sale – intermediaries like retailers and wholesalers. This method is usually adopted to sell industrial goods of high value and also goods like perishable commodities. In this type of selling, the marketing activities are performed by the producer himself.

2. Producer, retailer and consumer:

This is single phase distribution where the manufacturer sells the goods to retailer who in turn sells to the consumer. This is a popular method of distribution because of emergence of super markets and big departmental stores. The retailer procures the goods in large quantities from the manufacturer and sells them to the consumers.

3. Producer-wholesaler-retailer and consumer:

This is called two stage marketing where two intermediaries are involved. This is the traditional channel of distribution for the sale of consumer goods. This channel is most suitable for widely scattered markets.

4. Producer-distributor-wholesaler-retailer and consumer:

This type of distribution network is required when large number of retailers and wholesalers are present. Hence it becomes difficult for the producer to keep contact with such a large sales agencies. Hence the producer employs few distributors.

Usually the consumer goods are produced in large scale and everyone requires these goods. Hence a big channel of distribution is required whereas industrial goods are costly and few requirements are there. Hence a short channel of distribution.

Channel members

Distribution channels can thus have a number of levels. Kotler defined the simplest level that of a direct contact with no intermediaries involved, as the 'zero-level' channel.

The next level, the 'one-level' channel, features just one intermediary; in consumer goods a retailer, for industrial goods a distributor. In small markets (such as small countries) it is practical to reach the whole market using just one- and zero-level channels.

In large markets (such as larger countries) a second level, a wholesaler for example, is now mainly used to extend distribution to the large number of small, neighborhood retailers or dealers.

Channel functions and flows

Marketing channels are sets of interdependent organizations involved in the process of making a product or service available for use or consumption. You can think of a marketing channel as a kind of delivery system. The goal of the system is to move goods from producers to consumers. Achieving that goal depends on the smooth flow, backwards and forwards, of goods, information, and money. Each participant in the channel plays a role in that flow. Therefore, each participant has a direct effect on the efficiency of the whole system. The question is not whether goods, information, and money must be moved. The question is who should move them and how well can they do it.

Basically channel functions classifies as primary and secondary: **Primary function focuses on re**duce contacts, negotiate price, transport & Store product, handle promotions and secondary function focuses on financing, information and assuming risk of distribution. Jobbers typically go to small retailers, those with no big wholesalers. Multiple channels will have more distributors but high status retailer might not want same goods as middle or low level retailers.

4.7 FACTORS INFLUENCING CHANNEL OF DISTRIBUTION:

The following are the most important factors which influence channel of distribution:

1. Consumer needs : it depend on lot size in terms of how many units or packing
2. Centralization and decentralization of distribution that drive customer satisfaction
3. Delivery time which effect the customer waiting time
4. availability of variety of product as per the customer wants
5. Service expectations of customer across the channels of distribution

The factors influence the selection of channel are: customer characteristics, product attributes, type of organization, competition, marketing environmental forces and characteristics of intermediaries are all factors in selecting a distribution channel.

i) Nature of Goods:

The first and most factor that influences on the choice of type of channel of distribution is the nature of goods. Perishable goods like cake, breads and snakes are needed to the sold quickly are sold normally directly buy the manufacturers to the consumer through own retail outlets. Goods can be last longer can be handled by more intermediaries to insure a larger market.

ii) Size of the Market:

In order to ensure that their goods are marketed as widely as possible, producers who do not want be load with the problems of managing their own retail outlets normally sale their goods to wholesalers. Thus we see that bigger the market, the larger will be the channel of distribution.

iii) Quantity of Goods Bought:

Most producers are normally not willing to entertain small orders from small retailers, because of the large amount of paper work involved. However, orders from large retailer or wholesalers are normally large.

iv) Size of Firm Producing the Goods:

Very big firms, which have the financial, and human resources normally not only produce the goods but also setup their own retail outlets. Smaller sized producers may prefer to concentrate on the technical aspects of the production and leave the marketing of goods to other.

Channel decisions

The channel decision is very important. In theory at least, there is a form of trade-off: the cost of using intermediaries to achieve wider distribution is supposedly lower. Indeed, most consumer goods manufacturers could never justify the cost of selling direct to their consumers, except by mail order. Many suppliers seem to assume that once their product has been sold into the channel, into the beginning of the distribution chain, their job is finished. Yet that distribution chain is merely assuming a part of the supplier's responsibility; and, if they have any aspirations to be market-oriented, their job should really be extended to managing all the processes involved in that chain, until the product or service arrives with the end-user. This may involve a number of decisions on the part of the supplier:

- Channel membership
- Channel motivation
- Monitoring and managing channels

Channel membership

1. Intensive distribution - Where the majority of resellers stock the 'product' (with convenience products, for example, and particularly the brand leaders in consumer goods markets) price competition may be evident.

2. Selective distribution - This is the normal pattern (in both consumer and industrial markets) where 'suitable' resellers stock the product.

3. Exclusive distribution - Only specially selected resellers or authorized dealers (typically only one per geographical area) are allowed to sell the 'product'.

Channel motivation

It is difficult enough to motivate direct employees to provide the necessary sales and service support. Motivating the owners and employees of the independent organizations in a distribution chain requires even greater effort. There are many devices for achieving such motivation. Perhaps the most usual is 'incentive': the supplier offers a better margin, to tempt the owners in the channel to push the product rather than its competitors; or a competition is offered to the distributors' sales personnel, so that they are tempted to push the product. Dent defines this incentive as a Channel Value Proposition or business case, with which the supplier sells the channel member on the commercial merits of doing business together. He describes this as selling business models not products.

MONITORING AND MANAGING CHANNELS

In much the same way that the organization's own sales and distribution activities need to be monitored and managed, so will those of the distribution chain.

In practice, many organizations use a mix of different channels; in particular, they may complement a direct sales force, calling on the larger accounts, with agents, covering the smaller customers and prospects.

Conflict, cooperation, and competition

No matter how much thought a company gives to channel design, no matter how much effort it puts into creating efficient processes, conflict is inevitable. As long as channel members retain some degree of independence, there can never be a perfect match between the goals and priorities of all channel members. As long as channel relationships depend on the interpretation of written agreements, there will always be room for confusion over the rights and responsibilities of channel members.

Types of conflict

Conflict can crop up in a number of places. It can occur between different levels in a marketing channel (**Vertical Conflict**). Retailers might resent the power of distributors. Manufactures might feel that retailers are not supportive of a national promotional campaign.

Conflict can occur between parties at the same level in a channel (**Horizontal Conflict**). Retailers in one region might complain that retailers in another region enjoy unfair advantages. Or franchise holders might complain that the parent company is creating too many new franchises.

Finally, conflict can occur between channels in a multi-channel system (**Multi-Channel Conflict**). For example, a distributor might complain that direct sales are cutting into the traditional store-based market.

Managing channel conflict

Sometimes the only solution to conflict is the dissolution of a channel relationship. However, companies that take concrete steps to facilitate communication can often find ways to resolve disputes. Remember that channels are meant to benefit all members. Therefore, companies should do everything they can to develop strong relationships in which all channel members have confidence in the overall desirability of the channel and in which clear, common goals eases the resolution of conflict.

4.8 PHARMA DISTRIBUTION CHANNEL

In a geographically diverse and extremely competitive market where sales volumes are high, distribution plays a crucial role. Further, the common incidence of brand substitutions makes it imperative for a company to make available its brands at all times and at various levels of distribution.

The distribution channel for pharmaceutical products is as below:

Channels of Distribution

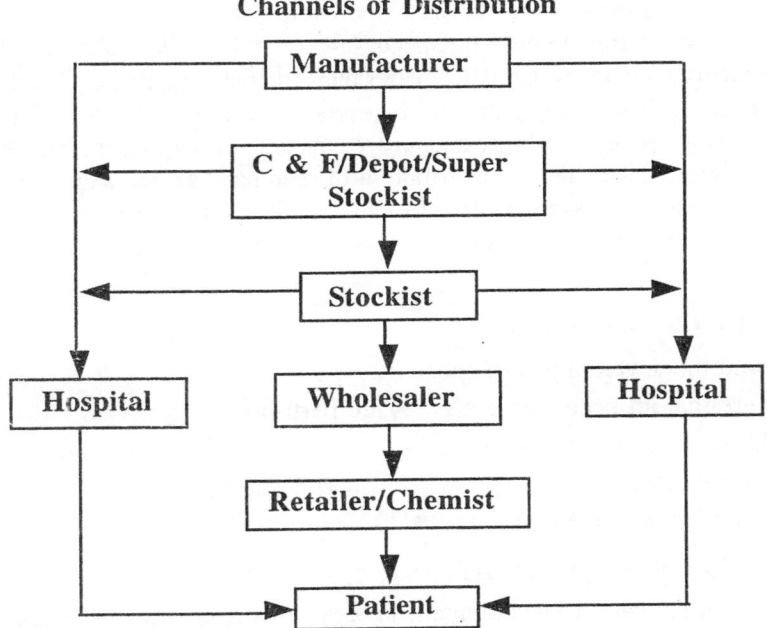

It is estimated that there are 60000 stockists and more than 550000 retailers in the country, plus the population of dispensing doctors. These doctors account for roughly 10 per cent of the pharma market. During the seventies and early eighties, there were few but large distributors. As the pharma companies expanded their marketing operations, these distributors faced logistic problems while attempting to cater to emerging markets. As a result of this, many small players became stockists and wholesalers, making the sector fragmented, and hence, more localized. According to the Retail Druggists and Chemists Association, there were roughly 10000 distributors and 125000 retail chemists in India in 1978. The number of distributors has increased six-fold, and retail outlets five-fold during the last two decades.

Drug distribution in India has been undergoing changes following liberalization. The changes have been initiated by pharma companies, which are increasingly replacing company owned depots and warehouses with Clearing and Forwarding (C and F) Agents. The aim is to curtail overheads. The C & F agents operate under contract   on companies' behalf. An agent is paid a fee that depends on the turnover of products, and ranges from 4 per cent on a high turnover product to 10 per cent on a low turnover product. Because of extended transit time, companies can move seasonal product well in advance to C and F agents without incurring ex-factory excise costs.

4.9 SALES ORGANIZATION

The sales management function represents an integral part of the marketing management function. The sales manager, therefore, is responsible for developing an effective Sales Organization in order to implement all aspects of the company's marketing plan. A sales organization is an organizational unit in Logistics that structures the company according to its sales requirements. Each sales organization represents a "selling unit" in the legal sense. Its responsibilities include product liability and any claims to recourse that customers may make. It is also responsible for the sale and distribution of merchandise and negotiates sales price conditions. Sales organizations can be used to reflect regional subdivisions of the market, for example by states. A sales transaction is always processed entirely within one sales organization.

Purpose of Sales Organization

- To permit the development of specialists
- To assure that all necessary activities are performed
- To achieve coordination or balance
- To define authority
- To economize on execution time

Sales organization development process

The Sales Organization Development Process entails creation of a specific pattern of work in which human and material resources can be utilized in the most efficient manner. Thus, the prime task of the sales manager is to develop a suitable organizational structure that will stimulate all employees toward effective performance.

Since the sales organization development process represents a continuous task that is carried out in a constantly changing environment, it is essential to ensure high flexibility of the **Sales Organizational Structure**.

Reasons for a flexible sales organizational structure

The basic Sales Organization Development Process entails four steps, as outlined below.

1. Determine the tasks that must be performed to implement the sales plan, e.g. forecasting, prospecting, selling, order taking.
2. Classify the tasks and group them into related sets of activities on the basis of product, customer, or sales territory requirements.

3. Assign set of activities to an individual position or positions.

4. Establish supervision and reporting relationships between positions.

Factors to be considered for sales organisation development:

1. One important consideration of the sales organization development process is the **Unity of Command Principle.** This principle suggests that each employee should report to only one person within the organization.

   This is a general principle that is particularly useful in the sales management environment. When employees report to more than one individual, they may be given contradicting instructions that can, in turn, cause ineffective performance. It is essential, therefore, to prevent such a condition to avoid confusion among sales employees.

2. Another issue that should be considered by the sales manager relates to the **Span Of Control**, or the number of subordinates that can be effectively supervised by one manager. The importance of this issue depends upon the size of the sales organization and is particularly critical for larger companies. Small and medium-sized organizations usually employ a moderate number of sales people and seldom experience problems caused by an excessive span of control.

3. The sales manager should also consider the issue of **Centralization or Decentralization of Control** over the company's sales activities.

   A small organization normally starts its operations from one office, and management exercises centralized control over sales force activities. When the organization grows and develops business relations with customers in different geographic locations, however, it may be useful to decentralize control over the sales force activities. This may require a branch to be opened in a suitable geographic location in order to ensure effective service of local customers.

   Decentralization of sales activities helps minimize the travel time and expenses incurred by sales people and maximize the quality of sales service provided by customers.

4. Finally, important consideration should be given by the sales manager to the issue of **Organizational Specialization.** Since companies build their activities around customer requirements, it is essential to develop a sales organization that will provide the most effective service in the marketplace. Several types of organizational specialization could be considered by the sales manager, as illustrated below.

Types of the sales organizational specialization

1. Geographic Specialization
2. Product Specialization
3. Customer Specialization
4. Functional Specialization

Geographically-specialized sales organization

Geographic Specialization is particularly suitable for an organization that operates in widespread geographic markets. In this type of organization, each sales person is assigned to sell all products to all customers within a specified geographic location. A typical structure of a **Geographically-Specialized Sales Organization** is illustrated below.

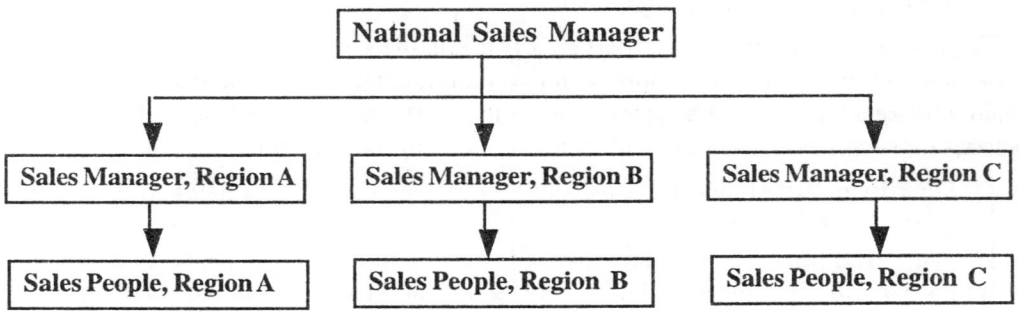

Main advantages and disadvantages of the geographically-specialized organization structure are outlined below.

GEOGRAPHICALLY-SPECIALIZED SALES ORGANIZATION	
Advantages	**Disadvantages**
One of the advantages of this structure is that it stimulates development of strong ties between sales people and their customers. In addition, travel time and selling costs can be substantially reduced because each sales person covers limited sales territory.	One of the disadvantages of this structure is that a particular sales person can handle only a limited number of un-complicated products or product lines.

Product-specialized sales organization

Product Specialization is generally used by industrial organizations that offer various lines of products to the market. This type of structure is effective in the distribution of different highly-technical products. In this type of organization, each sales person is trained to handle a particular product or product line. Thus, the number of sales people depends upon the variety of products handled by the organization. A typical structure of a Product-Specialized Sales Organization is illustrated below.

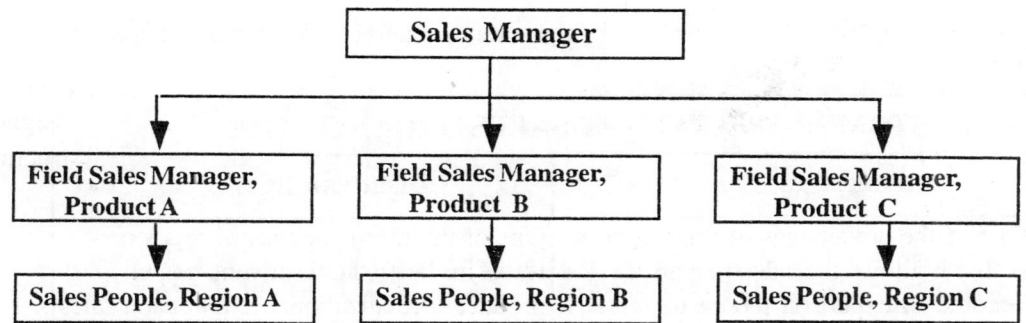

Main advantages and disadvantages of the product-specialized sales organization are outlined below.

PRODUCT-SPECIALIZED SALES ORGANIZATION	
Advantages	**Disadvantages**
One of the advantages of this structure is that it stimulates development of sound product knowledge by sales people. This, in turn, enables the company to provide an effective product and technical support to their customers.	One of the disadvantages of this structure is that each sales person must cover a much larger territory, which increases traveling time and selling expenses.

Customer-specialized sales organization

Customer Specialization is frequently used by organizations that offer their products to different industries. In this type of an organization, each sales person is assigned to a particular industry or individual customer. A typical Customer-Specialized Sales Organization structure is illustrated below.

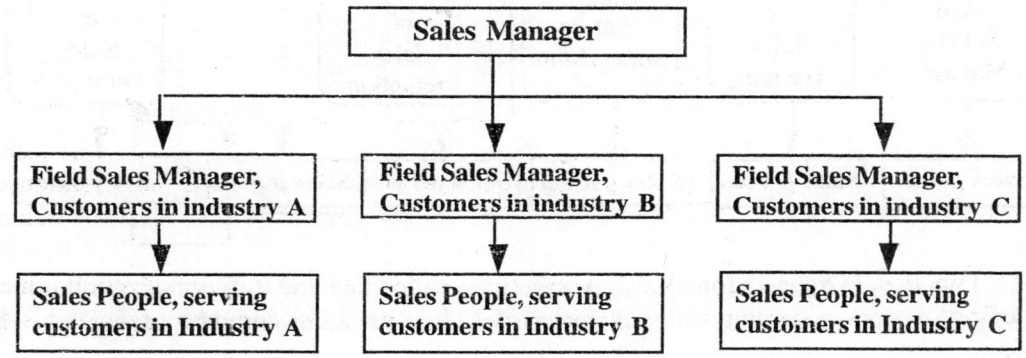

Main advantages and disadvantages of the customer-specialized sales organization are outlined below.

CUSTOMER-SPECIALIZED SALES ORGANIZATION	
Advantages	**Disadvantages**
One of the advantages of this structure is that it allows the sales person to become an expert on the customers operations and stimulates the development of strong company-customer relations	One of the disadvantages of this structure, similar to the disadvantages of product specialization, are that each sales person must cover a wide territory, spend more time on the road, and incur high selling expenses.

Function-specialized sales organization

Functional Specialization is most appropriate for organizations that offer relatively narrow product lines to non-segmented and geographically concentrated markets.

In this type of an organization, each sales person is assigned particular functional responsibilities for the entire range of customers. Two basic responsibilities are usually assigned to sales people in Function-Specialized Sales Organizations

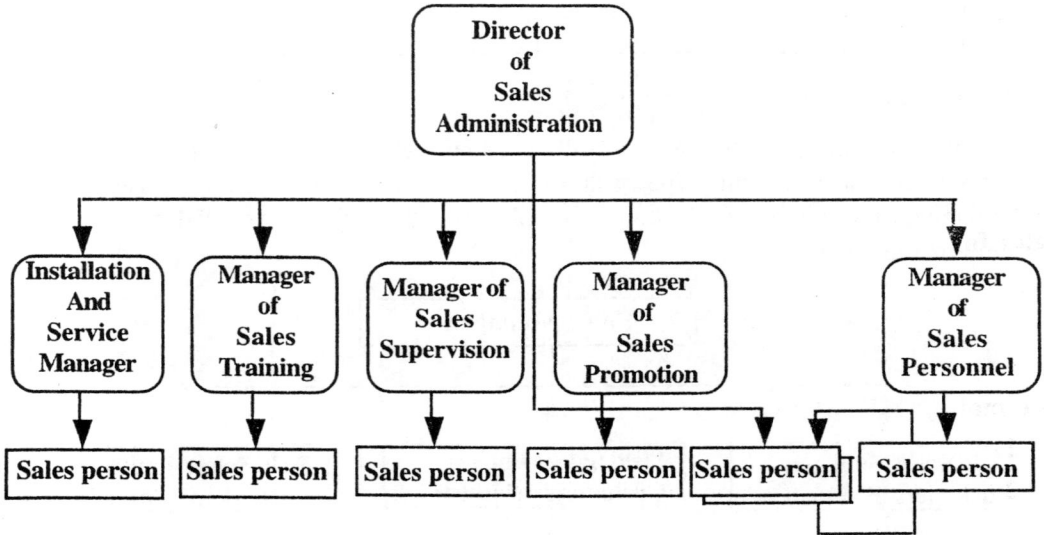

Functional Organizational Design sometimes called line and staff organization is the grouping of work according to its characteristics. It is the most common organizational design.

4.10 SALES PROMOTION

Sales promotion consists of diverse collection of incentive tools, mostly short term designed to stimulate quicker or greater purchase of particular product or services by consumers or the trade. Sales promotion is the process of **persuading a potential customer to buy the product**. It can be part of the personal selling process.

Sales promotion is a marketing discipline that utilizes a variety of incentive techniques to structure sales-related programs targeted to consumers, trade, and/or sales levels that generate a specific, measurable action or response for a product or service.

Sales promotion objectives:

The purpose of sales promotion is to stimulate consumer trial. Strengthen a long term relationship with retailer, reward loyal customers, increase repurchase rates of occasional users and to attract new users.

Consumers
- Encouraging large volume
- Building trial among non-users
- Attracting competitors customers

Retailers
- Persuading to carry new items
- Maintain higher level of inventory
- Encouraging off-season buying
- Offsetting competitors promotion
- Building brand loyalty
- Gaining entry into new retailers

Sales force
- Support of new product or model
- Stimulating off-season sales
- Encouraging new prospects

The main methods of sales promotion are:

1.   **Samples: A small amount of a product offered to consumers for trial.**

2.   **Money off coupons** – customers receive coupons, or cut coupons out of newspapers or a products packaging that enables them to buy the product next time at a reduced price.

3.   **Competitions** – buying the product will allow the customer to take part in a chance to win a prize (e.g. Coca Cola ring pulls).

4.   **Discount vouchers** – a voucher (like a money off coupon).

5.   **Cash refund offer (rebate):** offer to refund part of the purchase price of a product to consumers who send a proof of purchase to the manufacturer.

6.   **Free gifts** – a free product when buy another product.

7.   **Point of sales materials** – e.g. posters, display stands – ways of presenting the product in its best way or show the customer that the product is there.

8.   **Loyalty cards** – e.g. Nectar and Air Miles; where customers earn points for buying certain goods or shopping at certain retailers – that can later be exchanged for money, goods or other offers.

9.   Examples of recent sales promotions are: Tesco computers for schools, Cadbury's sport in the community and Café Nero free coffee card

10.   **Loyalty cards** have recently become an important form of sales promotion. They encourage the customer to return to the retailer by giving them discounts based on the spending from a previous visit.

11.   Loyalty cards can offset the discounts they offer by making more sales and persuading the customer to come back. They also provide information about the shopping habits of customers – where do they shop, when and what do they buy? This is very valuable marketing research and can be used in the planning process for new and existing products.

12.   **Premium:** Goods offered either free or at low cost as incentive to buy a product.

13.   **Patronage reward**: Cash or other award for the regular use of certain company's products or services (ex: airline frequent flier plans)

14.   **Cross promotion:** Use one brand to advertise another non competing brand

4.11 PHARMA MARKETING PROCESS AND ITS CHALLENGES

While many pharmaceutical companies have successfully deployed a plethora of strategies to target the various customer types, recent business and customer trends are creating new challenges and opportunities for increasing profitability. In the pharmaceutical and healthcare industries, a complex web of decision-makers determines the nature of the transaction (prescription) for which direct customer of pharma industry (doctor) is responsible. Essentially, the end-user (patient) consumes a product and pays the cost. Use of medical representatives for marketing products to physicians and to exert some influence over others in the hierarchy of decision makers has been a time-tested tradition. Typically, sales force expense comprises an estimated 15 percent to 20 percent of annual product revenues, the largest line item on the balance sheet. Despite this other expense, the industry is still plagued with some very serious strategic and operational level issues.

From organizational perspective the most prominent performance related issues are enlisted below:

- Increased competition and shortened window of opportunity.
- Low level of customer knowledge (Doctors, Retailers, Wholesalers).
- Poor customer acquisition, development and retention strategies
- Varying customer perception
- The number and the quality of medical representatives
- Very high territory development costs
- High training and re-training costs of sales personnel
- Very high attrition rate of the sales personnel
- Busy doctors giving less time for sales calls
- Poor territory knowledge in terms of business value at medical representative level.
- Unclear value of prescription from each doctor in the list of each sales person
- Unknown value of revenue from each retailer in the territory
- Virtually no mechanism of sales forecasting from field sales level, leading to huge deviations

MARKETING MODELS FOR PHARMA BUSINESS STRATEGY

1. **Super Core Model** involving the search for, and distribution of a small number of drugs from **Chronic Threapy Area** that achieve substantial global sales. The success of this model depends on achieving large returns from a small number of drugs in order to pay for the high cost of the drug discovery and development process for a large number of patients. Total revenues are highly dependant on sales from a small number of drugs.

2. **Core Model** in which a larger number of drugs from **Acute Threapy Area** are marketed to big diversified markets. The advantage of this model is that its success is not dependant on sales of a small number of drugs.

SUMMARY:

The mission of marketing is to satisfy customer needs. That takes place in a social context. In developed societies marketing is needed in order to satisfy the needs of society's members. Industry is the tool of society to produce products for the satisfaction of needs. Marketing mix consist of 4Ps which are the ideas to consider when marketing a product. They form the basis of the marketing mix. Getting this mix right is critical in order to successfully market a product. The 4Ps are: Product, Price, Promotion and Place.

The product life cycle plays and important role in marketing. Product life cycle is the course of a product's sales and profits over its lifetime. It involves five distinct stages: Product Development, Introduction, Growth, Maturity, and Decline. Depending on which stage the product is at in its lifecycle will determine which element of the 4P's will have the most emphasis. If the product is just being introduced, a different marketing strategy will be required compared to if it was in its decline stage.

Marketing channels (<u>Distribution</u> channels) move <u>goods</u> and services for producers to consumers. It overcomes the major time, place and possession gaps the separate good and services from those who would use them. Manufacturers, wholesalers, and retailers as well other channels members exist in channel arrangements.

A sales organization is an organizational unit in Logistics that structures the company according to its sales requirements. Each sales organization represents a "selling unit" in the legal sense. Its responsibilities include product liability and any claims to recourse that customers may make. It is also responsible for the sale and distribution of merchandise and negotiates sales price conditions. Sales organizations can be used to reflect regional subdivisions of the market, for example by states. A sales transaction is always processed entirely within one sales organization.

REVIEW QUESTIONS

1. What do you mean by Marketing? Explain the concept of societal marketing concept.

2. What is marketing mix? Explain with reference to pharma industry.

3. What are the various levels of channel of distribution?

4. What is Product Life Cycle (PLC). Suggest strategies to extend the product life cycle with examples.

5. What are channels of Distribution and its importance in market building?

6. What are the different factors to be considered while deciding on channels of distribution?

7. What is sales organization and what are the different types of sales organizations available in the marketing?

8. What is sales promotion? Explain the methods of sales promotion

9. What are the marketing models available in pharma industry? Explain the Pharma Marketing Process and its Challenges.

Chapter 5

PHARMA INDUSTRY

5.1 INTRODUCTION TO INDIAN PHARMACEUTICAL INDUSTRY

India is among the fastest growing pharmaceutical markets in the world. The domestic pharmaceutical market recorded sales of US$7.3 billion in 2006 with a growth of 17.5 per cent over the previous year. Of this, retail sales were US$6.2 billion, while institutional sales were estimated to be around US$1.2 billion.

The Indian pharmaceutical industry was estimated to be around US$13.2 billion in 2006-07. Of this, domestic consumption of pharmaceuticals accounted for nearly 57 per cent while

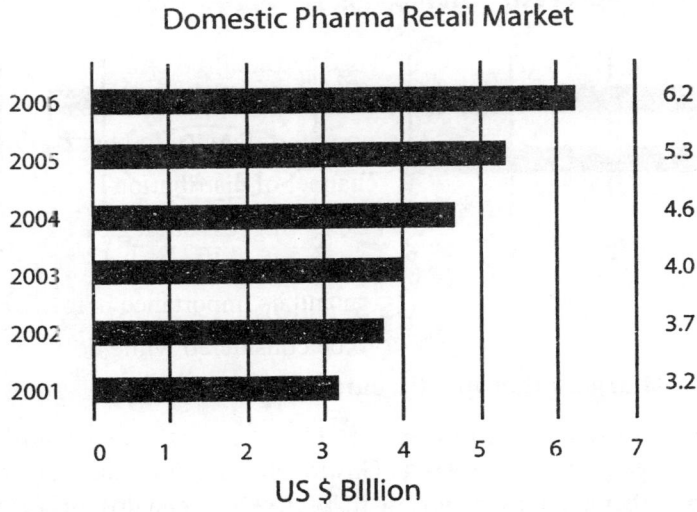

Domestic Pharma Retail Market

the rest 43 per cent was constituted by exports. The domestic market has grown at a composite CAGR of 9.5 per cent over the past five years.

However, in 2006, the market witnessed an accelerated growth of more than 17 per cent, primarily on account of increased clarity on tax reforms especially the Value Added Tax (VAT) implementation. In the long run, the market is expected to maintain a healthy growth rate of 12-13 per cent. It is expected to cross US$10 billion mark by 2010 and would reach US$12 to 13 billion approximately, by 2012.

BREAKUP OF SALES - INDIAN PHARMA INDUSTRY

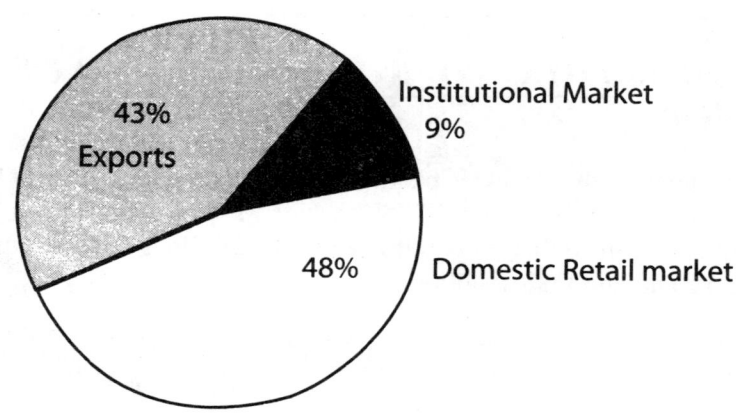

Forecasted Indian Pharmceutical Market

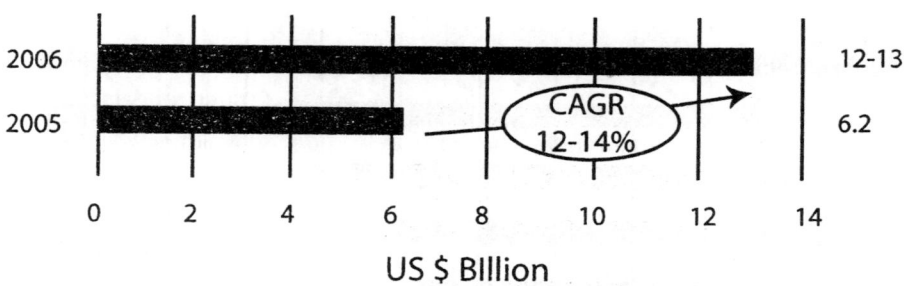

US $ BIllion

Anti Infectives – Largest therapeutic category:

Anti-infectives is the highest revenue earning segment with a contribution of 18 per cent to the total domestic sales in 2005-06. Gastro intestinal (GI) and cardiovascular are the 2nd and 3rd largest therapeutic categories, respectively. Cephalosporins, penicillin's and quinolones are key drug classes among anti-infectives, with a share of around 78 per cent of the country's anti-infectives market.

Market Share of Key Therapeutic Categories December 2006	
Anti - Infectives	18%
Gastrointestinal	11%
Cardiovascular	10%
Respiratory	9%
Vitamins/ Minerals	9%
Analgesics	9%
Gynaec	5%
CNS	5%
Dermatology	5%
Antidiabetic	4%
Others	13%

Elimentary and metabolism constituted around 25 per cent of the domestic formulation market in 2005-06 and grew by 10.7 per cent between 2003-04 and 2005-06. Oral anti-diabetics and anti-peptic ulculcerants are the fastest growing segments in this category.

Pharmaceutical Industry in India-Growth

- As per the present growth rate, the Indian Pharma Industry is expected to be a US$ 20 billion industry by the year 2015

- The Indian Pharmaceutical sector is also expected to be among the top ten Pharma based markets in the world in the next ten years

- The national Pharma market would experience the rise in the' sales of the patent drugs

- The sales of the Indian Pharma Industry would worth US$43 billion within the next decade

- With the increase in the medical infrastructure, the health services would be transformed and it would help the growth of the Pharma industry further
- With the large concentration of multi national pharmaceutical companies in India, it becomes easier to attract foreign direct investments
- The Pharma industry in India is one of the major foreign direct investments encouraging sectors

Role of Pharmaceutical Industry in India GDP-CRAMS

- The Indian Pharmaceutical Industry is one of fastest emerging international center for contract research and manufacturing services or CRAMS
- The main factors for the growth of the CRAMS is due to the international standard quality and low cost
- The estimated value of the CRAMS market in 2006 was US$895 million
- Indian already has the biggest number of US Food and Drug Administration (USFDA)
- standardized manufacturing units outside the territory of United States
- Around 50 more new manufacturing units are to be set up in accordance to the USFDA and UK Medicines and Healthcare Regulatory Agency (MHRA) standards
- With all these development India is posed to become the biggest producer of drugs in the world
- Some of the major domestic players in this sector are Paras Pharma, Bal Pharma, Unijules Life Sciences, Flamingo Pharma, Venus Remedies, Surya Organics and Chemicals, Centaur Pharma, Kemwell, Coral Labs
- The contract manufacturing market in India pertaining to the multinational companies is expected to worth US$900 million by the year 2010

Role of Pharmaceutical Industry in India GD-India Advantage

- India has the advantage of the cost, as the cost of labor, the cost of inventory is much lower than other places
- The multinational companies, investing in research and development in India may save up to 30% to 50% of the expenses incurred
- The cost of hiring a research chemist in the US is five times higher than its Indian counterpart
- The manufacturing cost of pharmaceutical products in India is nearly half of the cost incurred in US
- The cost of performing clinical trials in India is one tenth of the cost incurred in US

- The cost of performing research in India is one eighth of the cost incurred in US

With liberalization, globalisation and new obligations undertaken by India under the WTO Agreements, the drug and pharmaceutical industry in the country has been facing many new challenges. Accordingly, the Department has undertaken several policy initiatives in order to improve R&D conditions in the industry. The major policy being the **Drug Policy**, which has been announced and modified, from time to time, with the aim of achieving the following objectives:-

§   Ensuring abundant availability, at reasonable prices, of essential life saving and prophylactic medicines of good quality

§   Strengthening the system of quality control over drug and pharmaceutical production and distribution as well as promoting their rational use

§   Encouraging R&D in the pharmaceutical sector in a manner compatible with the country's needs and with particular focus on diseases endemic or relevant to India

§   Strengthening the indigenous capability for cost effective quality production and exports of pharmaceuticals by reducing barriers to trade in the sector and

§   Creating an environment conducive to channelising new investments into the pharmaceutical industry and to introducing new technologies and drugs.

GROWTH OF INDIAN PHARMACEUTICAL INDUSTRY

The Indian Pharmaceuticals sector has come a long way, being almost non-existing during 1970, to a prominent provider of health care products, meeting almost 95% of country's pharmaceutical needs. The domestic pharmaceutical output has increased at a compound growth rate (CAGR) of 13.7% per annum. Currently the Indian pharmaceutical industry is valued at approximately $8.0 billion. Globally, the Indian industry ranks 4th in terms of volume and 13th in terms of value. Indian pharmaceuticals industry has over 20,000 units. Around 260 constitute the organized sector, while others exist in the small scale sector.

GLOBAL PHARMA INDUSTRY AND CHALLENGES

The global pharma industry today is faced with two challenges: to develop and utilize scientific knowledge to derive new drugs and to do it at an affordable cost. The Indian pharma industry is well-positioned to address these twin challenges because of the vast availability of talented and skilled scientific manpower. The Rs.28,000 crore Indian pharma industry has been operating under a new world order from January 1 2005. From that date, in compliance with the prior commitment given under the WTO agreement the country has switched over to the product patent regime from the process patent regime that was in existence hitherto.

The main challenges facing the sector are the following.

- Growth in the domestic formulations market is slowing down.

- Domestic bulk drugs industry is facing intense competition due to cheap imports.

- Price wars between regional and local pharma companies are driving down prices, exerting pressure on margins.

- MNC pharma companies are getting more aggressive at protecting their patents and defending their market share after patent expiry.

- There has been considerable confusion in the grant of EMR, (Exclusive Marketing Rights) due to lack of transparency in the process.

    The huge domestic market (worth Rs.2,14,000 crore in 2002) with a billion plus population presents a tremendous opportunity to the Indian pharma industry though the growth is still in single digits. A roadmap for growth can be the following.

- Indian CROs (Clinical Research Organizations) have an opportunity to access the $6 billion (Rs.72,000 crore) global market for clinical trials which is expected to grow to over $0 billion by 2010.

- Indian pharma companies can focus on new drugs for neglected diseases like malaria, kala azar and tuberculosis, which are big killers in many developing countries.

- Indian pharma companies should reduce their dependence on the US market and explore promising markets like Europe and Japan. At $5 billion, Japan is the world's second largest pharmaceutical market after the US.

- Indian pharma companies can profitably tap the huge under-penetrated Chinese markets. By 2010, China will emerge as the fifth largest pharmaceutical market in the world with revenues of over $4 billion – three times its current size.

- The global herbal market is expected to grow to Rs.25,000 crore by 2010. India's share in this market currently is a dismal 5%The country with its traditional base has to grab a larger share of the market.

- Companies keen on exploiting process patents have an opportunity to operate in the least developed countries where product patent regime will not be operational till 2016.

- The R & D outsourcing market has grown from $.4 billion in 1997 to $.3 billion. Indian firms like Dr.Reddy's, Shasun, Suven & the Hyderabad based Divi's laboratories have already undertaken contract research for foreign majors.

- In-licensing global brands and selling them in the domestic market commands higher price margins of 15 to 18%

- The US generics market is definitely a high-risk high-reward game. To succeed, companies should identify products long before their patent expiry and complete regulatory work.

- With the advent of the product patent regime, Indian drug makers should diversify their process re-engineering skills towards advanced Novel Drug Delivery Systems (NDDS) and further into New Drug Discovery (NDD).

The Pharma Industry the world over is fragmented given the vast array of therapeutic groups specially segmented markets, and alternative configurations of value chain for various dosage forms. The structure of market is oligipolistic at the level of therapeutics and highly competitive for Over the Counter (OTC) and generic categories. The pharmaceutical industry worldwide is expected to grow between 6 and 8 per cent per annum during this decade or so. While price increases are responsible for nearly 60 per cent of this growth, while volume increases explain 25 per cent and sale of new drugs (sold at higher prices) result in 15 per cent of the growth. The generic component of the world Pharma market is expected to experience a boom in the current decade, which could substantially increase the export prospects of developing countries like India.

Production:

The production of pharmaceuticals reached US$296.4 billion in 1996. Of this, the OTC market accounted for US$48 billion and generics US $13.8 billion. The dominance of the developed countries, especially, the USA and Japan, and large multinational companies (MNCs) is quite striking in the global pharmaceutical production and trade. The USA is the largest producer of pharmaceuticals, accounting for nearly 28 per cent of the world pharmaceutical production. Japan accounts for about 18 per cent, Germany 8 per cent, France 7 per cent, the UK 3 per cent and Canada 2 per cent of the global production. India's share in world production is estimated at around one per cent.

The current value of world market for generics is estimated at US$30 billion. Of this, the USA accounts for US$12.3 billion, Western Europe US$7.13 billion and Japan US$5.1 billion. The remaining is accounted for by a large number of Asian and African countries. By 2003, the generic market is expected to reach US$43 billion with Japan, Europe and USA being the major markets. Among the world's largest 200 odd Pharma firms, 50 are Japanese and 33 are of US origin. Further the largest 50 companies produce 60 per cent of world output of drugs and pharmaceuticals as also cater to about half of the drug needs of the developing world. Interestingly, over the past two years, mergers and acquisitions worth more than US$1000 billion involving over 15 major companies have taken place worldwide.

RESEARCH AND DEVELOPMENT

The industry is also substantially dependent on research and development (R and D) on a continuous basis. Pharma industry is a typical case where R and D and profitability are closely interrelated. Increasingly, R and D have come to "dictate profitability" and the profitability, in turn, will govern the scale and scope of R and D expenditure. The need for firms to recoup the huge and growing costs of research and drug development has made protection of intellectual property rights an impending issue in the nineties. During the present decade of the 21st century, the challenge is likely to intensify once much of the differences/doubts over the issue of intellectual property rights (IPRs) are ironed out or clarified. The manifold widespread value chain and emerging possibilities in the spheres of production, marketing, distribution and R and D are opening up opportunities for firms to become specialised and focus on specific segments, molecules, dosage forms and areas of operation.

The pharmaceutical industry is a highly research and knowledge intensive industry mainly because of the need to sustain a pipeline of new drugs to replace old ones. On an average, large global companies in drugs and pharmaceuticals spend 12-15 per cent of their annual sales turnover on R and D. In the US, the ratio of R and D cost to sales turnover is estimated at 11.2 per cent, compared to 5 per cent for telecom, 4.2 per cent for automotive and an all industry composite of 3.8 per cent.

There has been a phenomenal increase in the cost of developing a new drug. In 1976 a new drug could be developed at the cost of about US$54 million (including capital and other indirect costs). By the beginning of the nineties this had escalated to US$59 million. From the concept to market a new drug has to go through a series of pre-clinical and clinical trials. It has been estimated that of the 5000 to 10000 substances screened, only 250 enter pre-clinical testing. From among these, approximately five enter the clinical testing phase and finally one drug gets approved. In order for the whole process to complete, it takes about 10 to 15 years.

The high investment and high risk involved in developing and commercialising a drug has posed major challenges to the pharmaceutical manufacturers who engage in basic research. This has led to the demand for strengthening intellectual property laws.

5.2 CURRENT STATUS AND ITS ROLE IN NATIONAL ECONOMY

With around 14%f annual growth the   **Pharmaceutical Companies** in India is worth USD 3.1 billion. It is the largest generic drugs producer in the world and has substantial contribution towards meteoritic growth of India Inc.

The pool of **'Pharmaceutical Company'** is dominated by generic manufacturers. Although, some first line companies are slowly shedding 'Generic' tag and dawning 'Innovator' tag to get a global footage, but still generic drugs accounts for 80%of revenue. 'Pharmaceutical Companies in India ' is getting technologically strong and self reliant. 'Pharmaceutical Companies in India ' are armed with:

- Low costs of production & R&D costs (around 70%ess than their Western counterparts).
- Highly innovative scientific manpower.
- Hosts of national and private laboratories.
- A strong IPR regime following WTO and WIPO norms.

Pharmaceutical Market in India is actively partnering with Government, NGOs and other Healthcare providers to improve the health and quality of life by innovating and developing safe, cost-effective and quality medicines. It also aims to increase the access of medicines to people in rural areas and those living at or below the poverty line. Companies like Ranbaxy, Dr. Reddy's Lab, Lupin Lab, Torrent Pharmaceuticals, Glenmark etc are performing excellently at the global level also. Ranbaxy has recently won a fierce battle against infringement (Norway) involving key Norwegian patents on Atorvastatin (a cholesterol-lowering drug marketed by Pfizer). MNC ' Pharmaceutical Companies in India ' are aggressively forging collaboration, acquisitions and even cross- licensing with foreign firms for greater reach, both in domestic and world market. 'Pharmaceutical Company in spite of registering fabulous growth is still laced with some negative market imperatives. Pharmaceutical Companies Operating in India ' is a pool representing about 250 large Pharmaceuticals manufacturers and suppliers and about 8000 Small Scale Pharmaceutical & Drug Units which forms the core (including 5 Central Public Sector Units).

The issues are:

- 'Patentable inventions' with respect to Sec 3 (d)of the Patents acts and Rules.
- Compulsory Licensing.
- Data Exclusivity.
- Spurious drugs.
- Availability.
- Price control of essential drugs.
- Sky high price of drugs manufactured by foreign companies.

To be one of the largest and most advanced in the world ' Pharmaceutical Market in India 'must address the issues of exporters, manufacturers and suppliers. ' Pharmaceutical Companies in India ' offers tremendous growth opportunities in years to come especially in the areas of Biological Sciences Research (particularly genomics and proteomics), Clinical Research & Development and Innovative Process Chemistry.

The pharmaceutical industry is the world's largest industry due to worldwide revenues of approximately US$.8 trillion. Pharma industry has seen major changes in the recent years that place new demands on payers, providers and manufacturers. Customers now demand the same choice and convenience from pharma industry that they find in other segment.Indian Pharmaceutical Industry is poised for high consistent growth over the next few years, driven by a multitude of factors. Top Indian Companies like Ranbaxy, DRL CIPLA and Dabur have already established their presence.

The pharmaceutical industry is a knowledge driven industry and is heavily dependent on Research and Development for new products and growth. However, basic research (discovering new molecules) is a time consuming and expensive process and is thus, dominated by large global multinationals.

The Indian pharmaceutical industry came into existence in 1901, when Bengal Chemical & Pharmaceutical Company started its maiden operation in Calcutta. The next few decades saw the pharmaceutical industry moving through several phases, largely in accordance with government policies. Commencing with repackaging and preparation of formulations from imported bulk drugs, the Indian industry has moved on to become a net foreign exchange earner, and has been able to underline its presence in the global pharmaceutical arena as one of the top 35 drug producers worldwide. Currently, there are more than 2,400 registered pharmaceutical producers in India. There are 24,000 licensed pharmaceutical companies. Of the 465 bulk drugs used in India, approximately 425 are manufactured here. India has more drug-manufacturing facilities that have been approved by the U.S. Food and Drug Administration than any country other than the US. Indian generics companies supply 84% of the AIDS drugs that Doctors without Borders uses to treat 60,000 patients in more than 30 countries

The Indian pharmaceutical industry currently tops the chart amongst India's science-based industries with wide ranging capabilities in the complex field of drug manufacture and technology. A highly organized sector, the Indian pharmaceutical industry is estimated to be worth $4.5 billion, growing at about 8 to 9 percent annually. It ranks very high amongst all the third world countries, in terms of technology, quality and the vast range of medicines that are manufactured. It ranges from simple headache pills to sophisticated antibiotics and complex cardiac compounds, almost every type of medicine is now made in the Indian pharmaceutical industry.

The Indian pharmaceutical sector is highly fragmented with more than 20,000 registered units. It has expanded drastically in the last two decades. The **Pharmaceutical and Chemical industry in India** is an extremely fragmented market with severe price competition and government price control. The **Pharmaceutical industry in India** meets around 70%f the country's demand for bulk drugs, drug intermediates, pharmaceutical formulations,

chemicals, tablets, capsules, orals and injectibles. There are approximately 250 large units and about 8000 Small Scale Units, which form the core of the pharmaceutical industry in India (including 5 Central Public Sector Units).
India has the following advantages:

- **Competent workforce:** India possess a skillful work force with high managerial and technical competence.

- **Cost-effective chemical synthesis:** The track record for development, particularly in the area of improved cost-beneficial chemical synthesis for various drug molecules is excellent.

- **Legal & Financial Framework:** India is a democratic country with a solid legal framework and strong financial markets. There is already an established international industry and business community.

- **Information & Technology:** It has a good network of world-class educational institutions and established strengths in Information Technology.

- **Globalization:** The country is committed to a free market economy and globalization. Above all, it has a 70 million middle class market, which is constantly growing.

- **Consolidation:** After many years, the international pharmaceutical industry has discovered great opportunities in India. The process of consolidation, which has become a popular phenomenon in the world pharmaceutical industry, has started taking place in the **Indian pharmaceutical industry** as well. The **Indian pharmaceutical industry** which is worth US $3.1 billion is growing at the rate of 14 percent per annum.

5.3 ROLE OF PHARMA INDUSTRY TO INDIAN ECONOMY

The **Role of Pharmaceutical Industry in India GDP** is immense. For the past few years the Indian Pharmaceutical Industry is performing very well. The varied functions such as contract research and manufacturing, clinical research, research and development pertaining to vaccines are the strengths of the Pharma Industry in India. Multinational pharmaceutical corporations outsource these activities and help the growth of the sector. The Indian Pharmaceutical Industry has a bright future.

Role of Pharmaceutical Industry in India GDP-Facts

- The Pharmaceutical Industry in India is one of the largest in the world
- It ranks 4th in the world, pertaining to the volume of sales
- The estimated worth of the Indian Pharmaceutical Industry is US$6 billion
- The growth rate of the industry is 13% per year

- Almost most 70% of the domestic demand for bulk drugs is catered by the Indian Pharma Industry
- The Pharma Industry in India produces around 20% to 24% of the global generic drugs
- The Indian Pharmaceutical Industry is one of the biggest producers of the active pharmaceutical ingredients (API) in the international arena
- The Indian Pharma sector leads the science-based industries in the country
- The pharmaceutical sector has the capacity and technology pertaining to complex drug manufacturing
- Around 40% of the total pharmaceutical produce is exported
- 55% of the total exports constitute of formulations and the other 45% comprises of bulk drugs
- The Indian Pharma Industry includes small scaled, medium scaled, large scaled players, which totals nearly 300 different companies
- There are several other small units operating in the domestic sector

The Indian drugs and pharmaceutical industry, over the years, has shown tremendous progress in terms of infrastructure development, technology base creation as well as product usage. On the global platform, India holds fourth position in terms of volume and thirteenth position in terms of value of production in pharmaceuticals. The pharmaceutical industry has been producing bulk drugs belonging to all major therapeutic groups requiring complicated manufacturing processes as well as a wide range of pharma machinery and equipments. It has also developed excellent 'good manufacturing practices' (GMP) compliant facilities for the production of different dosage forms. Besides, the amendment to the Patents Act, 1970 [enactment of Patents (Amendment) Act, 2005], has opened up new avenues for the sector. The new patent regime has ushered in the era of product patents for the pharmaceutical sector, in line with the obligations under the **World Trade Organisation (WTO)** and **Trade-Related Aspects of Intellectual Property Rights (TRIPS) Agreement**. As a result, the Indian pharmaceutical industry has become self-reliant in several areas and has developed a more sound and technologically advanced R&D segment.

Indian pharma industry: SWOT analysis

It is often said that the pharma sector has no cyclical factor attached to it. Irrespective of whether the economy is in a downturn or in an upturn, the general belief is that demand for drugs is likely to grow steadily over the long-term. True in some sense. But are there risks? This article gives a perspective of the Indian pharma industry by carrying out a SWOT analysis (Strength, Weakness, Opportunity, Threat).

Before we start the analysis lets look a little back in the industry's last six years performance. The Industry is a largely fragmented and highly competitive with a large number of players having interest in it. The following chart shows the breakup of the growth (YoY) of Indian pharmaceutical industry in last six years. The SWOT analysis of the industry reveals the position of the Indian pharma industry in respect to its internal and external environment.

Strengths:

1. Indian with a population of over a billion is a largely untapped market. In fact the penetration of modern medicine is less than 30% in India. To put things in perspective, per capita expenditure on health care in India is US$ 93 while the same for countries like Brazil is US$ 453 and Malaysia US$189.

2. The growth of middle class in the country has resulted in fast changing lifestyles in urban and to some extent rural centers. This opens a huge market for lifestyle drugs, which has a very low contribution in the Indian markets.

3. Indian manufacturers are one of the lowest cost producers of drugs in the world. With a scalable labor force, Indian manufactures can produce drugs at 40% to 50% of the cost to the rest of the world. In some cases, this cost is as low as 90%.

4. Indian pharmaceutical industry posses excellent chemistry and process reengineering skills. This adds to the competitive advantage of the Indian companies. The strength in chemistry skill help Indian companies to develop processes, which are cost effective.

Weakness:

1. The Indian pharma companies are marred by the price regulation. Over a period of time, this regulation has reduced the pricing ability of companies. The NPPA (National Pharma Pricing Authority), which is the authority to decide the various pricing parameters, sets prices of different drugs, which leads to lower profitability for the companies. The companies, which are lowest cost producers, are at advantage while those who cannot produce have either to stop production or bear losses.

2. Indian pharma sector has been marred by lack of product patent, which prevents global pharma companies to introduce new drugs in the country and discourages innovation and drug discovery. But this has provided an upper hand to the Indian pharma companies.

3. Indian pharma market is one of the least penetrated in the world. However, growth has been slow to come by. As a result, Indian majors are relying on exports for growth. To put things in to perspective, India accounts for almost 16% of the world population while the total size of industry is just 1% of the global pharma industry.

4. Due to very low barriers to entry, Indian pharma industry is highly fragmented with about 300 large manufacturing units and about 18,000 small units spread across the country. This makes Indian pharma market increasingly competitive. The industry witnesses price competition, which reduces the growth of the industry in value term. To put things in perspective, in the year 2003, the industry actually grew by 10.4% but due to price competition, the growth in value terms was 8.2% prices actually declined by 2.2%

Opportunities

1. The migration into a product patent based regime is likely to transform industry fortunes in the long term. The new patent product regime will bring with it new innovative drugs. This will increase the profitability of MNC pharma companies and will force domestic pharma companies to focus more on R&D. This migration could result in consolidation as well. Very small players may not be able to cope up with the challenging environment and may succumb to giants.

2. Large number of drugs going off-patent in Europe and in the US between 2005 to 2009 offers a big opportunity for the Indian companies to capture this market. Since generic drugs are commodities by nature, Indian producers have the competitive advantage, as they are the lowest cost producers of drugs in the world.

3. Opening up of health insurance sector and the expected growth in per capita income are key growth drivers from a long-term perspective. This leads to the expansion of healthcare industry of which pharma industry is an integral part.

4. Being the lowest cost producer combined with FDA approved plants, Indian companies can become a global outsourcing hub for pharmaceutical products.

Threats:

1. There are certain concerns over the patent regime regarding its current structure. It might be possible that the new government may change certain provisions of the patent act formulated by the preceding government.

2. Threats from other low cost countries like China and Israel exist. However, on the quality front, India is better placed relative to China. So, differentiation in the contract manufacturing side may wane.

3. The short-term threat for the pharma industry is the uncertainty regarding the implementation of VAT. Though this is likely to have a negative impact in the short-term, the implications over the long-term are positive for the industry

5.4 PSU'S IN PHARMA INDUSTRY

There are five public sector undertakings (PSUs) in the pharmaceutical sector, namely:-

§   **Indian Drugs and Pharmaceuticals Ltd. (IDPL)**

§   **Hindustan Antibiotics Ltd. (HAL)**

§   **Bengal Chemicals and Pharmaceuticals Ltd. (BCPL)**

§   **Bengal Immunity Ltd. (BIL)**

§   **Smith Stanisteet Pharmaceuticals Ltd.(SSPL)**

Two of the four pharmaceutical PSUs - Rajasthan Drugs and Pharmaceuticals (RDPL) and Hindustan Antibiotics (HAL) - are getting into the fast-growing segment of anti-retroviral (ARV) drugs, which are used in the treatment of AIDS.

The entry of the PSUs into this market, estimated at Rs 3,000 crore a year, is certain to bring down the prices as the PSUs intend to price their drugs 20%heaper than the prevailing market rates.There is already a downward pressure on the prices of ARVs as a result of Gilead Sciences, the US-based multi-national, entering into as many as seven licensing agreements with Indian companies to make and market its ARV, tenofovir.

The imminent entry of the two PSUs in the ARV segment is part of the plan to revive them. All the four pharma PSUs - the other two being Indian Drug & Pharmaceuticals and Bengal Chemicals & Pharmaceuticals - are sick. Chances are that IDPL and BCPL will also join the ARV fray.

Announcing this, Union minister for chemicals & fertilisers Ram Vilas Paswan said RDPL would launch six ARVs and HAL another three.

The HIV-infected population in India touched an alarming 5.7 million in 2005. While RDPL and HAL have already starting producing ARVs for the first line treatment and received approvals for good manufacturing practices, the companies will soon be file for registration with World Health Organisation and pre-qualification, following which they can export to other countries as well.

The department of chemicals and petrochemicals has already put in place a 'preferred procurement policy' for 102 pharmaceutical formulations exclusively from pharma PSUs and their subsidiaries, for a period of five years. With the total central and state purchases through the bulk procurement scheme of Rs 3,500-4,000 crore, pharma PSUs are expected to secure 10%f this pie.

Health ministry invests 14 crore to PSU vaccine units

The Union Health Ministry has launched serious efforts, including approval of funds, to revive the three Public Sector Vaccine (PSV) manufacturing units. The Health Ministry has approved the proposal to invest around Rs 14 crore in the Central Research Institute at Kasauli in Himachal Pradesh, as recommended by an oversight committee. The panel had prepared the roadmap for revamping the manufacturing facility at CRI and submitted to the DGHS.

Karnataka Antibiotics and Pharmaceuticals Ltd (KAPL) and Rajasthan Drugs and Pharmaceuticals Ltd (RDPL) are doing well. Bengal Chemicals and Pharmaceuticals Ltd and Uttar Pradesh Drugs and Pharmaceuticals Ltd are on the revival mode.

Hindustan Antibiotics Ltd (HAL) and Indian Drugs and Pharmaceuticals Ltd (IDPL) - are in the process of completely shutting shop.

5.5 MANUFACTURE OF BASIC DRUGS, SYNTHETIC AND DRUGS OF VEGETABLE ORIGIN:

The pharmaceutical industry includes the manufacture, extraction, processing, purification, and packaging of chemical materials to be used as medications for humans or animals. Pharmaceutical manufacturing is divided into two major stages: the production of the active ingredient or drug (primary processing, or manufacture) and secondary processing, the conversion of the active drugs into products suitable for administration. This document deals with the synthesis of the active ingredients and their usage in drug formulations to deliver the prescribed dosage.

Formulation is also referred to as galenical production. The main pharmaceutical groups manufactured include:

- Proprietary ethical products or prescriptiononly medicines (POM), which are usually patented products

- General ethical products, which are basically standard prescription-only medicines made to a recognized formula that may be specified in standard industry reference books

- Over-the counter (OTC), or nonprescription, products.

The products are available as tablets, capsules, liquids (in the form of solutions, suspensions, emulsions, gels, or injectables), creams (usually oil-in-water emulsions), ointments (usually waterin- oil emulsions), and aerosols, which contain inhalable products or products suitable for external use. Propellants used in aerosols include chlorofluorocarbons (CFCs), which are being phased out. Recently, butane has been used as a propellant in externally applied products.

The major manufactured groups include

- Antibiotics such as penicillin, streptomycin, tetracyclines, chloramphenicol, and antifungals

- Other synthetic drugs, including sulfa drugs, antituberculosis drugs, antileprotic drugs, analgesics, anesthetics, and antimalarials

- Vitamins

- Synthetic hormones

- Glandular products

- Drugs of vegetable origin such as quinine, strychnine and brucine, emetine, and digitalis glycosides

- Vaccines and sera

- Other pharmaceutical chemicals such as calcium gluconate, ferrous salts, nikethamide, glycerophosphates, chloral hydrate, saccharin, antihistamines (including meclozine, and buclozine), tranquilizers (including meprobamate and chloropromoazine), antifilarials, diethyl carbamazine citrate, and oral antidiabetics, including tolbutamide and chloropropamide

- Surgical sutures and dressings

The principal manufacturing steps are (a) preparation of process intermediates; (b) introduction of functional groups; (c) coupling and esterification; (d) separation processes such as washing and stripping; and (e) purification of the final product. Additional product preparation steps include granulation; drying; tablet pressing, printing, and coating; filling; and packaging. Each of these steps may generate air emissions, liquid effluents, and solid wastes.

BASIC DRUGS AND PHARMACEUTICALS

The drugs and pharmaceuticals industry has made considerable progress in the last two decades. The production of basic drugs and pharmaceutical formulations was estimated to be Rs. 226 crores and Rs. 1150 crores respectively in 1979-80. The contribution 01 the public sector amounted to 26 per cent in the case of bulk drugs and 6.3 per cent in the case of formulations, the organised private sector accounting for 63.4 per cent and 67 per cent respectively with the balance being the output of the small industry sector. To meet the supply gap, bulk drugs worth Rs. 150 crores (landed cost) were imported.

Requirements of bulk drugs and formulations by 1984-85 have been estimated at Rs. 815 crores and Rs. 2450 crores respectively. The production of basic drugs is expected to increase to Rs. 665 crores and the balance of Rs. 150 crores would continue to be met by imports. The production of basic drugs in public sector is expected to increase from Rs. 59 crores to Rs. 215 crores and formulations from Rs. 72 crores to Rs. 330 crores.

The policy on drugs aims at:

a. development of self-reliance in drug technology;

b. providing a leadership role to the public sector;

c. making drugs available at reasonable prices and in abundance to meet the health needs of the people; and

d. fostering and encouraging the growth of the Indian sector.

Keeping in view the important role assigned to the public sector, a provision of Rs. 145 crores has been made for Hindustan Antibiotics Ltd., Indian Drugs and Pharmaceuticals Ltd. and the three drug units in the Eastern region: Smith Stanstreet Pharmaceuticals Ltd., Bengal Chemical & Pharmaceutical Works Ltd., and Bengal Immunity Co. Ltd.

The major on-going schemes which would be completed are: the second phase expansion of the synthetic drugs plant; the nicotinamide project and expansion of the antibiotics plant of IDPL and thp expansion of the streptomycin and penicillin plant of HAL. A number of joint sector units are proposed to be established with the participation of State Governments to serve local needs. Provision has also been made for new starts in the Plan on a selective basis.

Drug development is a blanket term used to define the entire process of bringing a new drug or device to the Market. It includes Drug discovery / product development, pre-clinical research (micro organisms/animals) and Clinical trials (on humans). Few people still refer to the drug development as mere preclinical development.

Synthetic sources

At present majority of drugs used in clinical practice are prepared synthetically, such as aspirin, oral antidiabetics, antihistamines, amphetamine, chloroquine, chlorpromazine, general and local anaesthetics, paracetamol, phenytoin, synthetic corticosteroids, sulphonamides and thiazide diuretics.

Advantages of synthetic drugs are:

•   They are chemically pure.

•   The process of preparing them is easier and cheaper.

•   Control on the quality of the drug is excellent.

•   Since the pharmacological activity of a drug depends on its chemical structure and physical properties, more effective and safer drugs can be prepared by modifying the chemical structure of the prototype drug

Drugs are obtained from the following natural sources

Oils . They are liquids which are insoluble in water. They are of three types and are used for various medicinal purposes.

i) *Essential Oils (or volatile oils):* Essential oils are obtained from leaves or flower petals by steam distillation, and have an aroma.

- They have no caloric or food value.
- They do not form soaps with alkalies.
- They do not leave greasy stain after evaporation.
- On prolonged stay, they do not become rancid (foul smell).
- They are frequently used as carminatives and astringents in mouth-washes.
- Some of these oils are solid at room temperature and sublime on heating e.g. menthol and camphor.
- Other examples are clove oil, peppermint oil, eucalyptus oil and ginger oil.

ii) *Fixed oils* are glycerides of stearic, oleic and palmitic acid.

- They are obtained from the seeds that are present within the cells as crystals or droplets.
- They are non-volatile and leave greasy stains on evaporation.
- They have caloric or food value.
- They form soaps with alkalies.
- On prolonged stay, they become rancid.
- They do not have marked pharmacological activity and have little pharmacological use except castor oil (purgative) or arachis oil (demulcent).
- They may be of vegetable origin e.g. olive oil, castor oil, croton oil and peanut oil or of animal origin e.g. cod liver oil, shark liver oil and lard .

5.6 EXPORT AND IMPORT TRENDS

Market trends

The industry has enormous growth potential. Factors listed below determine the rising demand for pharmaceuticals.

- The growing population of over of a billion
- Increasing income
- Demand for quality healthcare service
- Changing lifestyle has led to change in disease patterns, and increased demand for n ew medicines to combat lifestyle related diseases.

Demand for drugs for treatment of lifestyle-related diseases such as diabetes, cardiovascular diseases, and central nervous system are on the increase. There are around 700,000 new cases of cancer each year and total of around 2.5 million cases. It is estimated that there are around 40 million people in India with diabetes and the number is rising, 5.1 million HIV/AIDS patients, and 14 million tuberculosis cases. According to industry reports, while the Indian pharmaceutical industry witnessed a growth of 7 percent, the cardio-vascular segment recorded 15 to 17 percent growth and anti-diabetes segment of over 10-12 percent growth.

Historically, the low cost of domestically produced drugs together with government controlled prices, and the absence of patent regulations had made the market less attractive for foreign players. With the new patent laws in place the market scenario will change. Indian market will become attractive for foreign companies.

Import Market

According to contacts and industry studies, imports are estimated at 10 to 12 percent of the total market. The major suppliers are Switzerland, China, USA, Germany, Italy, Denmark, France, and UK. Imports include raw materials and finished products. Some major pharmaceuticals being imported include Provitamins and Vitamins, Cortisones, Hydrocortisone, Insulin, Penicillin, Osetrogen, Progesterone and other hormones, Erythromycin and other antibiotics, Antisera & other blood fraction, and Glycosides.

COMPETITION

Competition is mainly from the domestic manufacturers and imports from China because of the low manufacturing cost. With the new patent regulations the industry expects to see a major structural shift with the entry of foreign pharmaceutical manufacturers.

There are five government-owned companies the Indian public sector. These companies are

1. Indian Drugs and Pharmaceuticals,
2. Hindustan Antibiotics Limited,
3. Bengal Chemicals and Pharmaceuticals Limited,
4. Bengal Immunity Limited and
5. Smith Stanistreet Pharmaceuticals Limited.

Some of the major Indian private companies are

1. Alembic Chemicals,
2. Aurobindo Pharma,
3. Ambalal Sharabhai Limited,

4. Cadila Healthcare,
5. Cipla,
6. Dr. Reddy's,
7. IPCA Laboratories,
8. Jagsonpal Pharma,
9. J.B. Chemicals,
10. Kopran,
11. Lupin Labs,
12. Lyka Labs,
13. Nicholas Piramal,
14. Matrix Laboratories,
15. Orchid Chemical and Pharmaceuticals,
16. Sun Pharmaceuticals,
17. Ranbaxy Laboratories,
18. Torrent Pharma,
19. TTK Healthcare,
20. Unichem Labs and
21. Wockhardt.

The foreign companies in India include

1. Abott India,
2. Astra Zeneca India,
3. Aventis Pharma India,
4. Burrough-Wellcome,
5. Glaxo SmithKline,
6. Merck India,
7. Novartis,
8. Pfizer Limited and
9. Wyeth Ledele India.

India also exports pharmaceuticals to numerous countries around the world, including to the U.S., Germany, France, Russia and UK.

End Users

Around three quarters of the pharmaceuticals are for the retail market, rest for direct sales to the hospitals and nursing homes. End users of pharmaceuticals are the government and private healthcare service providers, and retailers. In India, healthcare service is provided both by the government (public) and private sector. The size of the Indian healthcare delivery market is estimated at $8.7 billion. The private sector provides for 63 percent of the healthcare market. With only 15 percent of the population covered by insurance, a large proportion of the healthcare spending is out of pocket spending.

Hospitals	16,000
Medical Colleges	171
Beds	870,161
Physicians	503,900
Nurses	737,000
Retail Chemists(Pharmacists)	500,000

Source: National Health Policy 2002, and Organization of Pharmaceutical Producer of Indian, and Espicom report

The government healthcare infrastructure includes primary health centers and sub centers in the villages that are the first point of contact that provide basic drugs for minor ailments. At the secondary level, the district hospitals and the community healthcare centers, and finally, at the tertiary level are the government owned hospitals and medical colleges. The private healthcare providers consist of private practitioners, for profit hospitals and nursing homes, and charitable hospitals. They are numerous and fragmented.

Market Access

Regulatory offices

The Central Drug Standard Control Organization (CDSCO) in the Ministry of Health is responsible for regulating pharmaceuticals in India, CDCSO's functions:

- Establish the drug standards and regulations, and administer the Drugs and Cosmetics Act

- Co-ordinate with the Drug Controllers in the states and union territories

- Approve import/manufacturing/sale of new drugs in India

- Check and control the quality of imported and manufactured pharmaceuticals

- It is the Central License Approving Authority with respect to blood and blood products, intravenous fluids, sera and vaccines.

Other organizations under the Ministry of Health and their functions include:

- The Central Drugs Laboratory, Kolkata, is responsible for testing samples of imported drugs. It is the designated laboratory under the Drugs and Cosmetics Act, and for samples referred by drug inspectors. It also supplies the reference standards for various drugs to pharmaceutical manufacturers.

- The Central Indian Pharmacopoeia Laboratory in Ghaziabad undertakes experimental work related to standards for drugs included in the Indian Pharmacopoeia and functions as a government analyst for several Indian states.

- The Central Drug Testing Laboratory in Chennai and in Mumbai, test drug samples and assist the CDSCO in the analysis of drug formulations and substances.

- The Drugs Consultative Committee is a statutory advisory body under the Drugs and Cosmetics Act that issues licenses to import biological and other special products.

- The Central License Approving Authority (CLAA) under the Drugs Controller General of India (DGCI) examines applications for licenses with respect to blood banks, sera, and vaccine under the Drugs and Cosmetics Act.

Market share of MNCs and Local companies

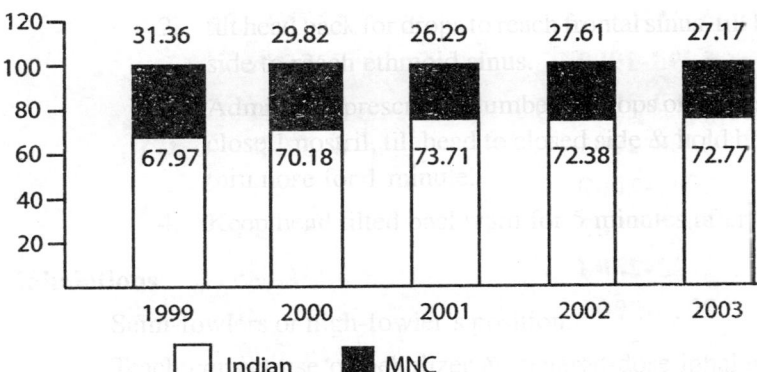

The exports constitute almost 40% of the total production of pharmaceuticals in India. India's pharmaceutical exports are to the tune of $.5bn currently, of which formulations contribute nearly 55% and the rest 45% comes from bulk drugs.

The export revenue now contributes almost half of the total revenue for the top 3 pharma majors: Dr Reddy's, Ranbaxy and Cipla. The other major exporters are Wockhardt Limited, Sun Pharmaceutical Industries Ltd. and Lupin Laboratories. The formulations and exports are largely to developing nations in CIS, South East Asia, Africa, and Latin America. In the last 3 years generic exports to developed countries have picked up.

Exports of Drugs, Pharmaceuticals and fine chemicals

1999-2000	2000-2001	2001-2002	2002-2003	2003-2004
Rs. 7230.16cr ($.60 bn)	Rs. 8757.47cr ($.95 bn)	Rs. 9834.7cr ($.18 bn)	Rs. 11925.4cr ($.65 bn)	Rs. 14100.00cr ($.13 bn)

Growth of pharmaceutical exports

1999-2000	2000-2001	2001-2002	2002-2003	2003-2004
15.57%	20.73%	11.13%	21.2%	18.24%

The country is also showing excellent performance on the Pharma export front. The figures of exports under this category during the current decade have been:

Pharma exports touched a level of over Rs. 24942 crores during 2006-07. Exports constitute a substantial part of the total production of Pharmaceuticals in India. Another note worthy feature of export is more of dosage form export to advanced markets like Europe, US, CIS Africa etc. The trend of exports is as follows: -

YEAR	EXPORT (Rs. in Crores)
1998-1999	6256.06
1999-2000	7230.16
2000-2001	8757.47
2001-2002	9751.20
2002-2003	12826.10
2003-2004	15213.24
2004-2005	17857.80
2005-2006	22578.98
2006-2007	24942.00

(Source:-Directorate General of Commercial Intelligence and Statistics --DGCIS, Kolkata)

TRADE

Allopathic Medicines:

Over the years the drugs and pharmaceuticals sector has emerged as a net foreign exchange earner, a status it has maintained since 1988-89. The average annual growth rate of exports between 1980-81 and 1998-99 was about 33 per cent as against 22 per cent in the case of imports. The ratio of exports to imports rose from 0.61 to 2.15 between the early 1980s and the end of 1990s. Finished formulations dominate the export kitty, while bulk drugs and chemicals dominate the import basket.

Region-wise breakup of Global Pharmaceutical Market (Global Size: $363 bn.):

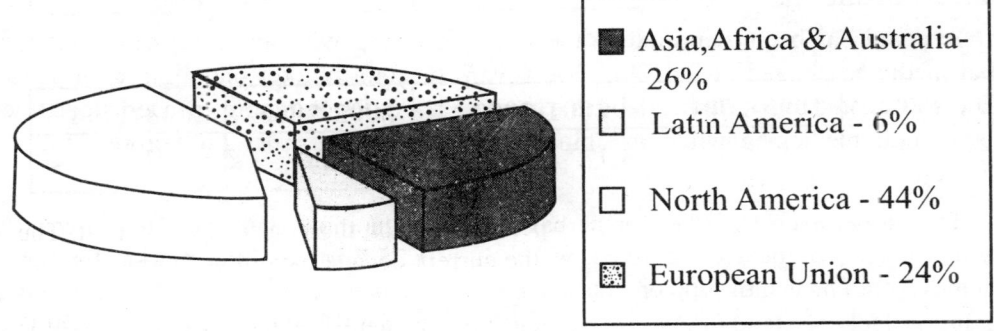

- Asia,Africa & Australia- 26%
- Latin America - 6%
- North America - 44%
- European Union - 24%

(Source: Indian Pharmaceutical Industry – Update, April 2003.)

The Indian manufacturers are increasingly tapping the export market. Export revenues now contribute almost half the total revenues for the top 3-Pharma majors, viz, Dr.Reddy's, Ranbaxy and Cipla. In financial year 01, exports constituted 38% of the total production of pharmaceuticals in India. The industry exported drugs worth Rs.87 bn, of which formulations contributed nearly 55% and the rest was from the bulk drugs. During the year, exports grew by 21% per year. In financial year 03, the Indian Pharma market is estimated to have exported drug worth Rs. 110 bn. The comparative advantage lies in the low cost of bulk drug manufacturers. In the past five years, the Pharma exports grew by 30% per annum. Formulation exports (i.e. finished products) are largely to developing nations in CIS, South East Asia, Africa and Latin America. In the last three
countries have picked up. In the coming years, opening up of US generics market and anti-AIDS market in Africa would keep export growth high.

In financial year 01, India's pharmaceuticals imports were approximately Rs.20.3bn. In the past five years, imports have registered a CAGR of only 2%. Imports of bulk drugs have slowed down because there is over capacity in the domestic market and the quality of bulk drugs manufactured by the domestic manufacturers has improved significantly.

Indian pharmaceutical exports are to the tune of Rs. 250 crores, of which nearly 50% are bulk drugs. It has been growing @ 20% per annum. The competitive pressure and DPCO has led the Pharma Industry to focus on export markets. In exports, domestic companies have a 3 – branched advantage over MNCs:

- Process Patents give freedom to make MNCs patented products, thus enabling wide therapeutic reach,

- Strong R&D and low manufacturing cost and

- No restrictions on export markets by patents' overseas ventures.

Ayurvedic Medicine:

Ayurved has been identified as the fastest growing with the organised market for Herbal medicine pegged at Rs.10bn. However, the total market including unorganised market is estimated to Rs.20bn. India is exporting about Rs.400 crores of Herbals extracts and Ayurvedic medicines, while on China's export is more than Rs.2000 crores in herbal medicines.

The global export market for herbal medicines is about $5bn, and is projected to cross $16 bn, in the next three years, which is just 25% of the total market for herbal medicines including health supplements and beauty products. The problem that the industry is facing is lack of standardization. Indian Government has understood the need for standardization and hence GMP has been introduced in this sector too. While government is doing its bit, the corporate sector seems to tap the export market by building the brands on global map.

The world exports of pharmaceuticals have been growing at a compound rate of about 13 per cent per annum from US $ 14.4 billion in 1983 to US $ 35 billion in 1993 and to about US $ 50 billion currently. Developed countries account for over 90 per cent of the world exports and 70 per cent of imports. The share of developing countries in world exports is about 5 to 7 per cent. China, Hong Kong, Singapore, Republic of Korea and India are the major exporters among developing countries.

The industry offers several opportunities for investments and trade owing to the following advantageous features:-

§   Self-reliance displayed by the production of 70 per cent of bulk drugs and almost the entire requirement of formulations within the country;

§   Low cost of production of quality bulk drugs and formulations

§   Low R&D costs

§   Strong scientific, innovative and technical manpower

▪   Excellent and world-class national laboratories specialising in process development and development of cost effective technologies

▪   Increasing balance of trade in pharma sector

▪   Efficient and cost effective source for procuring generic drugs, especially the drugs going off patent in the next few years

§   Excellent centre for clinical trials in view of the diversity in population

§   Fast growing biotech industry which has great potential in the international market

§   Apart from its strengths in manufacturing and exporting allopathic medicines, the systems of medicines like Ayurveda, Unani, Siddha, Yoga, Naturopathy and Homeopathy are also prevalent in the country.

Driven by all such factors, India has been recognized as one of the leading global players in pharmaceuticals. The annual turnover of the industry is estimated to be about US $17 billion (over Rs.68,000 crores) during 2006-07. Indian exports are destined to more than 200 countries around the globe including highly regulated markets of US, Europe, Japan and Australia. The value of exports of drugs and pharmaceuticals has increased   to

Rs. 4,942 crores in 2006- 07 from around Rs. 22,216 crores in 2005-06. While, the imports of medicinal and pharmaceutical products have been around Rs.5867.3 crores (provisional) in the year 2006-07. It is estimated that by the year 2010, the industry has the potential to achieve over Rs. 1,00,000 crore in formulations and bulk drug production. Moreover, increasing number of Indian pharmaceutical companies have been getting international regulatory approvals for their plants from agencies like USFDA (USA), MHRA (UK), TGA (Australia), MCC (South Africa), Health Canada, etc. India has the largest number of USFDA approved plants for generic manufacture. Leading Indian companies are now seeking more Abbreviated New Drug Approvals (ANDAs) in USA in specialized segments like anti infectives, cardiovasculars and central nervous system groups.

5.7 EXPORT AND IMPORT TRADE

The impact of the wide range of policy reforms post-1991 on drugs and pharmaceuticals trade is an issue that has been discussed widely. This discussion has also been linked to the debate sparked off by the changes in the patent regime that was expected to adversely affect the generic producers dominating the Indian pharmaceutical industry. It was argued that introduction of the product patent regime would restrict the generic producers' scope of operations, particularly their ability to export to preferred destinations. Imports would get a fillip not merely because of the restricted scope of operation of the domestic producers, but also because of the parallel process of lowering of tariffs. Furthermore, the removal of the ratio parameter, which insisted on local production to some extent and abolition of restrictions on foreign firms were expected to encourage imports of pharmaceutical products into India.

Variation in the Estimates

We would initiate the discussion by comparing the available estimates on India's pharmaceutical trade. The table below shows data from different sources for the latest years for which data are available from both industry and government sources.

Table 1: Export and Import of Drugs and Pharmaceuticals

(Rupees in crore)

	2003-04		2004-05		2005-06	
	Export	Import	Export	Import	Export	Import
Department of Chemicals and Petrochemicals, Ministry of Chemicals and Fertilizers (Annual Report 2006-07)	7445.0	1150.0	9263.0	1303.0	10821.0	1945.0
Department of Chemicals and Petrochemicals (http://chemicals.nic.in/pharma1.htm	15213.0	—	17857.0	—	22116.0	—
Report of Working Group on Drugs and Pharmaceuticals for the Eleventh Five Year Plan, Planning Commission of India	15213.2	2956.6	17857.8	3169.4	21579.0	4515.2
IDMA (45th Annual Publication, 2007)	15213.2	2956.6	17857.8	3169.4	21579.0	4515.2
OPPI (Indian Pharmaceutical Industry: Fact Sheet – 2005)	—	—	—	—	19800.0	4800.0
BDMA (www.bdmai.org)	14324.2	5085.0	16681.0	5630.0	—	—
Difference between lowest and highest figures (%)	104.3	342.2	92.8	332.1	104.4	146.8

There are huge differences in the figures provided by the different sources referred to in Table 1. For example, in 2004-05, the lowest estimates for both exports and imports were provided by the Department of Chemicals and Petrochemicals. While the Indian Drug Manufacturer's Association (IDMA) and the Working Group on Drugs and Pharmaceuticals for the Eleventh Plan provided the highest estimate for exports, the Bulk Drug Manufacturer's Association (BDMA) provided the highest estimates for imports. It is the magnitude of difference between the highest and the lowest estimates that are particularly significant.

In case of exports, the magnitude of exports of pharmaceutical products reported by the Department of Chemicals and Petrochemicals was only one half of that reported by the IDMA and the Working Group on Drugs and Pharmaceuticals for the Eleventh Plan. The difference between the lowest and highest estimates in case of imports was considerably larger. BDMA reported a figure that was more than three times larger than that provided by the Department of Chemicals and Petrochemicals. The fact that the trade figures given in the Annual Report of the Department of Chemicals and Petrochemicals are substantially different from the trade figures given in the website of the Department of Chemicals and Petrochemicals and in the Report of the Working Group on Drugs and Pharmaceuticals for the Eleventh Five Year Plan shows the magnitude of the lack of understanding of the issue even at the official level.

Figures provided by different industry sources are also at variance, particularly in respect of imports. There is a striking difference between the figures of BDMA on the one hand and IDMA or OPPI on the other. The difference was 42% in 2003-04 and it increased to 44% in 2005-06. A plausible explanation of the difference in the figures provided by the BDMA and OPPI-IDMA is the following.

In India there is a highly competitive bulk drug industry spreading across large, medium and small scale sectors. These producers largely depend on imported intermediates to process them into bulk drugs[1]. And BDMA, being an association of the producers of bulk drugs in the large, medium and small scale sectors, covers a larger number of production units as compared to IDMA or OPPI whose membership do not include the smaller producers. This may explain why the import figures of BDMA are larger than the figures of all other sources.

Trade data given in the Report of the Working Group on Drugs and Pharmaceuticals for the Eleventh Five Year Plan, which is sourced from DGCIS, is substantially different (99.4% difference in exports and 132.1% difference in imports) from the data given in the Annual Report of the Department of Chemicals and Petrochemicals, which has also seemingly sourced the data from DGCIS.

Trade quantities and values of these products are the same as given by the DGCIS. Exports add up to Rs9714.41 crore and imports to Rs8846.1 crore. However, the values of total exports and imports given in the same publication were very different - Rs11925 crore exports and Rs1102.5 crore imports. Thus it comes out that there are serious problems with the aggregate trade data given by industry associations as well. In this confusing scenario, it may be wise for one to collect data at the level of individual items to arrive at the aggregate trade figures.

Table 2: Exports and Imports of Drugs and Pharmaceuticals
(In US$ Million)

1990-91	316.5	641.7	-325.2
1991-92	424.6	470.8	-46.2
1992-93	411.9	497.3	-85.4
1993-94	589.7	682.1	-92.4
1994-95	736.1	1149.4	-413.3
1995-96	911.6	1489.2	-577.6
1996-97	1055.9	1493.2	-437.3
1997-98	1207.3	1500.1	-292.8
1998-99	1133.1	1166.1	-33.0
1999-00	1343.4	1398.7	-55.4
2000-01	1614.0	1338.2	275.8
2001-02	1733.3	1544.2	189.2
2002-03	2226.3	1906.3	320.1
2003-04	2324.8	2171.1	153.6
2004-05	2767.5	3034.6	-267.1
2005-06	3250.8	3746.5	-495.8
2006-07	4076.3	4516.1	-439.8
G.R 91-92 to 06-07	18.0	15.3	
G.R 91-92 to 99-00	18.4	12.5	
G.R 00-01 to 06-07	17.5	18.9	

Source: India Trades, CMIE.
Note: G.R – Average Annual Growth Rate

Table 3: Exports, Imports and Balance of Trade of Intermediates, Bulk Drugs and Formulations

(In US$ Million)

	Intermediates & Bulk Drugs*			Bulk Drugs**			Formulations			Other Drugs and Pharma Products		
	Exp	Imp	BoT	Exp	Imp	BoT	Exp	Imp	BoT	Exp	Imp	BoT
1990-91	56.3	488.0	-431.9	177.1	91.6	85.5	66.9	51.3	15.6	16.3	10.6	5.6
1991-92	126.0	360.0	-234.4	90.3	49.2	41.1	197.6	52.6	144.9	10.6	8.5	2.1
1992-93	130.0	423.0	-293.1	69.8	17.0	52.8	201.3	46.8	154.5	11.1	10.8	0.3
1993-94	164.0	619.0	-454.6	104.0	16.8	87.3	306.4	36.0	270.4	15.0	10.5	4.5
1994-95	233.0	1081.0	-848.1	113.9	21.1	92.8	373.9	31.1	342.7	15.1	15.8	-0.7
1995-96	306.0	1386.0	-1080.6	96.3	21.1	75.2	494.6	46.4	448.2	15.0	35.3	-20.4
1996-97	383.0	1429.0	-1045.5	123.9	10.6	113.4	528.6	38.4	490.3	20.0	15.5	4.5
1997-98	426.0	1377.0	-951.2	134.0	19.0	115.0	608.3	70.8	537.6	39.1	33.3	5.8
1998-99	403.0	1031.0	-627.2	133.5	18.9	114.6	577.7	87.4	490.3	18.4	29.2	-10.8
1999-00	486.0	1260.0	-773.5	174.1	24.8	149.3	661.2	83.6	577.6	21.6	30.4	-8.7
2000-01	667.0	1187.0	-520.0	150.6	27.9	122.7	754.7	92.9	661.8	41.4	30.1	11.3
2001-02	674.0	1377.0	-702.7	188.7	28.5	160.2	836.3	94.3	742.1	33.9	44.3	-10.4
2002-03	823.0	1668.0	-845.0	276.7	25.0	251.6	1090.6	161.4	929.2	36.3	52.1	-15.8
2003-04	704.0	1921.0	-1217.1	218.9	20.6	198.2	1356.7	178.2	1178.5	45.6	51.6	-6.0
2004-05	707.0	2745.0	-2038.1	352.2	23.7	328.5	1648.7	210.2	1438.5	60.0	55.9	4.1
2005-06	807.0	3306.0	-2499.4	207.5	27.0	180.4	2185.5	329.3	1856.2	50.8	83.8	-33.0
2006-07	900.0	3873.0	-2972.1	304.8	29.3	275.5	2800.1	492.7	2307.5	70.9	121.6	-50.7
G.R 91-92 to 06-07	21.9	16.5		8.9	-0.3		31.1	19.3		16.3	24.7	
G.R 91-92 to 99-00	30.9	15.2		4.2	-2.9		37.2	10.0		10.9	25.5	
G.R 00-01 to 06-07	10.3	18.1		14.9	3.2		23.1	31.2		23.1	23.8	

Source: India trades, CMIE.

Note: * bulk drugs of single chemical substance; ** bulk drugs of two or more chemical substances

India's balance of trade in drugs and pharmaceuticals has been negative from 1990-91 onwards except for the first four years of this millennium. Growth rates show that exports grew at 18.0% per annum and imports at 15.3% per annum from 1991-92 to 2006-07. In order to capture the impact of the new patent regime, the period of analysis has been divided into two—the period till 1999-2000 and the period from 1999-2000. Though the new patent regime came into being only in January 2005, the monopoly rights of the inventor had been protected from 1999 onwards through the Exclusive Marketing Rights (EMRs) provisions of the first amendment of the Indian Patents Act 1970. EMRs brought with them a five-year, patent-like monopoly for products covered by the product patent applications made under the mailbox system. The company securing the EMR has the exclusive rights to sell or distribute the article or substance covered in a patent application in a country. The 1999 amendment is an important first step towards enabling domestic legislation and institutions to provide for product patent rights in pharmaceuticals. The impact of the change in patent rights in exports and imports is expected to be felt from 1999-2000. The break-up of the period shows that the rates of growth of exports has declined marginally during the post-1999-00 period and imports has increased from 12.5% per annum during the pre-1999-00 period to 18.9% in the post-1999-00 period. Though this seems to support the argument that exports will decline and imports will increase, one has to look at data at a more disaggregated level for arriving at more meaningful conclusions.

Table 3 gives drugs and pharmaceutical products at a more disaggregated level. These products are classified into four broad categories––intermediates and bulk drugs, bulk drugs, formulations (including vaccines) and others. It is seen that India has consistent trade surpluses in two categories—bulk drugs and formulations. Of the remaining two categories, the balance of trade is consistently negative for intermediates and negative for most of the period for other drugs and pharmaceutical products. On the exports front, the bulk drugs, and other drugs and pharmaceutical products grew at higher rates during the post-1999-00 period as compared to the period before. But, these two groups account for only 9.2% of the total drugs and pharmaceuticals exported in 2006-07. The growth in the export of the other two groups, which account for 90.8% of the total exports, has declined in the period after 1999-00. The decline in the growth of exports for the two categories is definitely a cause for concern. The trends in imports are more alarming. The import of three categories of drugs and pharmaceuticals—intermediates and bulk drugs, bulk drugs and formulations—which account for 97.3% of total imports, have grown at higher rates in the post-1999-00 period. The growth was highest in the category of formulations; it increased by 21.2 percentage points.

Trade Policy

Most of the items under drugs and pharmaceuticals products are falling under HS code 30. They can be imported freely by paying the specified custom duties. In few cases the imports are subject to Wild Life (Protection) Act, 1971 and CITES.

Industry Policy

Industries under drugs and pharmaceuticals have to obtain an industrial licence to manufacture, since it falls under Annexure II which includes the list of industries for which industrial licensing is compulsory under Industries (Development & Regulation) Act, 1951.

Industrial undertakings are free to select the location of a project.

Entrepreneurs are required to obtain Statutory clearances relating to Pollution Control and Environment for setting up an industrial project. In respect of bulk drugs and pharmaceuticals, pesticides etc. environmental clearance needs to be obtained from the Ministry of Environment, Government of India. Items reserved for the small scale sector with investment of less than Rs. 10 million was also exempt from obtaining environmental clearance from the Central Government.

FDI up to 100 per cent is permitted on the automatic route for manufacture of drugs and pharmaceutical, provided the activity does not attract compulsory licensing or involve use of recombinant DNA technology, and specific cell / tissue targeted formulations.

FDI proposals for the manufacture of licensable drugs and pharmaceuticals and bulk drugs produced by recombinant DNA technology, and specific cell / tissue targeted formulations will require prior Government approval.

100 per cent Export Oriented Units (EOUs) and units in the Export Processing Zones (EPZs)/Special Economic Zones(SEZs), enjoy a package of incentives and facilities, which include duty free imports of all types of capital goods, raw material, and consumables in addition to tax holidays against export.

Tariff-non-tariff Policy

Maximum custom duty on any item falling under the code 30 is 56.83 per cent. This includes 30 per cent basic duty, 16 per cent additional duty and 4 per cent special additional duty. A lower 20 per cent basic duty is imposed if the imports are from preference areas. There are many items where additional duty is nil. A total 27 restricted items are there under the code 30 which require import license.

SUMMARY

India is among the fastest growing pharmaceutical markets in the world. The domestic pharmaceutical market recorded sales of US$ 7.3 billion in 2006 with a growth of 17.5 per cent over the previous year. Of this, retail sales were US$ 6.2 billion, while institutional sales were estimated to be around US$ 1.2 billion. Drugs and pharmaceuticals have generally reported that the Indian pharmaceutical industry is performing extremely well on the exports front. The growth rates of import of almost the entire drugs and pharmaceuticals (intermediates & bulk drugs, bulk drugs and formulations accounting for 97.3% of imports) have increased in the post 1999-00 period. Basic steps in manufacture of basic drugs, synthetic and drugs of vegetable origin are dealt. The role of pharma industry in development of Indian economy is presented. Subsequently further discussion is made on balance of payments.

REVIEW QUESTIONS

1. Explain the growth of Pharmaceutical industry in recent times in India?

2. Discuss the role of Pharma industry in building national economy and national health?

3. What is the future prospects of Pharma industry in India?

4. Analyze the SWOTs of India pharma market

5. Describe the Basic drug and vegetables drug development in India pharma?

6. Discuss the market trends in the Pharma exports and Imports?

Chapter 6

INSURANCE AND PHARMA

6.1 INTRODUCTION

Pharmaceuticals drugs are drugs given under the advice of doctors to cure various disorders. 70% of the country's demand for drugs, chemicals, capsules etc is met by these companies. In India there are about 250 large pharmaceutical manufacturers and about 8000 small scale pharmaceutical manufacturers. The total worth of Pharmaceutical industries is said to be about around $ 4 million and it is said to be growing at a rate of 10 to 12% annually.

Current Position of Indian Pharmaceutical Industries

Earlier when medical science had not made so much progress people used to go to vaids, who gave them medicines mostly made from plants and other herbal products. But the growing complexities of life made way for newer kind of physical disorders and to cure them hospitals and pharmaceutical industries also came up. Today you can find medicine for the simplest to the most complex physical disorders. Indian pharmaceutical industries have quality producers and today there are many international companies collaborated with India pharma Industries. The 250 large pharmaceutical companies have control of nearly 70% of the market and there is stiff price competition. Any drug approved by the Drug control Authority can be produced by the pharmaceutical companies and the low cost of production, development in science and technology, strength of national laboratories help the companies in their production.

Prospects of Pharmaceutical Industries in India

Some of the leading pharmaceutical companies of India are Ranbaxy, Sun, Pharma, Dr. Reddy's etc. Mixture of right product is very essential for the growth of the pharma companies. It also needs to take advantage of recent developments in biotechnology and information technology. Growth also depends on the fact how well these companies make their product and distributes them. Another thing which the Indian pharma companies have to improve is the research and development and they have to invest largely on research and development.

6.2 INTRODUCTION TO INSURANCE

Insurance is a mean to remove the hindrance of risk. risk factor is reduced by insurance. There are life insurance, fire insurance, marine insurance, car insurance, medical insurance and many more insurance facility given by insurance companies

The Indian Insurance sector is having a dream run. Today people have become very conscious about their future and so they are spending nearly 6 times on life insurance than they did before. The number of life insurance policies in India is the largest in the world and this sector contributes nearly 4 % in the GDP. The Indian insurance companies recorded a growth nearly 20% in premium in dollar terms, compared to the world market growth rate 0f only 3%.

Steps Taken by Government to Promote Insurance Sector

According to a study, the life insurance market premiums is likely to be around US$100 billion by 2012, and its contribution to GDP is likely to rise by 6%. The general Insurance Company has also grown to nearly 12% in 2007. Meanwhile the government has also taken few measures to boost this industry. Some of such measures are:

- FDI up to 26% has been permitted.

- Some state governments have also taken the initiatives to promote this sector. The government of Andhra Pradesh has decided to issue health cards to 18 million people living below poverty lines. As a result nearly 60 million people of the state will have insurance cover.

6.3 MAJOR FOREIGN INSURANCE COMPANIES IN INDIA

Many of the foreign companies are also coming to India. Global giants such as New York Life, Tokyo Marine, UK based prudential have formed joint ventures with many Indian companies. Some of the major joint venture companies are Bajaj Allianz, HDFC Standard, Aviva Life Insurance, Birla Sunlife, Met Life, Royal Sundaram etc.

The domestic insurance industry is believed to be around US$ 61 billion by 2010 and non- life insurance market is estimated to be around US$25 billion. The booming Insurance sector is sure to grow further in the coming years and it can be said that in the next few years, the Insurance sector in India will be on the top of the world insurance market.

Insurance companies

Insurance companies may be classified into two groups:

- *Life* insurance companies, which sell life insurance, annuities and pensions products.

- *Non-life*, *General*, or *Property/Casualty* insurance companies, which sell other types of insurance.

General insurance companies can be further divided into these sub categories.

- Standard Lines
- Excess Lines

In most countries, life and non-life insurers are subject to different regulatory regimes and different tax_ and accounting rules. The main reason for the distinction between the two types of company is that life, annuity, and pension business is very long-term in nature — coverage for life assurance or a pension can cover risks over many decades. By contrast, non-life insurance cover usually covers a shorter period, such as one year.

In the United States, standard line insurance companies are "mainstream" insurers. These are the companies that typically insure autos, homes or businesses. They use pattern or "cookie-cutter" policies without variation from one person to the next. They usually have lower premiums than excess lines and can sell directly to individuals. They are regulated by state laws that can restrict the amount they can charge for insurance policies.

Excess line insurance companies (aka Excess and Surplus) typically insure risks not covered by the standard lines market. They are broadly referred as being all insurance placed with non-admitted insurers. Non-admitted insurers are not licensed in the states where the risks are located. These companies have more flexibility and can react faster than standard insurance companies because they are not required to file rates and forms as the "admitted" carriers do. However, they still have substantial regulatory requirements placed upon them. State laws generally require insurance placed with surplus line agents and brokers not to be available through standard licensed insurers.

Insurance companies are generally classified as either ***mutual*** or *stock* companies. Mutual companies are owned by the policyholders, while stockholders (who may or may not own policies) own stock insurance companies. ***Demutualization*** of mutual insurers to form stock companies, as well as the formation of a hybrid known as a mutual holding company, became common in some countries, such as the United States, in the late 20th century. Other possible forms for an insurance company include ***reciprocals***, in which policyholders 'reciprocate' in sharing risks, and Lloyds organizations.

Reinsurance companies are insurance companies that sell policies to other insurance companies, allowing them to reduce their risks and protect themselves from very large losses. The reinsurance market is dominated by a few very large companies, with huge reserves. A reinsurer may also be a direct writer of insurance risks as well.

Captive Insurance companies may be defined as limited-purpose insurance companies established with the specific objective of financing risks emanating from their parent group or groups. This definition can sometimes be extended to include some of the risks of the parent company's customers. In short, it is an in-house self-insurance vehicle. Captives may take the form of a "pure" entity (which is a 100%subsidiary of the self-insured parent company); of a "mutual" captive (which insures the collective risks of members of an industry); and of an "association" captive (which self-insures individual risks of the members of a professional, commercial or industrial association). Captives represent commercial, economic and tax advantages to their sponsors because of the reductions in costs they help create and for the ease of insurance risk management and the flexibility for cash flows they generate. Additionally, they may provide coverage of risks which is neither available nor offered in the traditional insurance market at reasonable prices.

The types of risk that a captive can underwrite for their parents include property damage, public and product liability, professional indemnity, employee benefits, employer's liability, motor and medical aid expenses. The captive's exposure to such risks may be limited by the use of reinsurance.

Captives are becoming an increasingly important component of the risk management and risk financing strategy of their parent. This can be understood against the following background:

- heavy and increasing premium costs in almost every line of coverage;
- difficulties in insuring certain types of fortuitous risk;
- differential coverage standards in various parts of the world;
- rating structures which reflect market trends rather than individual loss experience;
- insufficient credit for deductibles and/or loss control efforts.

There are also companies known as 'insurance consultants'. Like a mortgage broker, these companies are paid a fee by the customer to shop around for the best insurance policy amongst many companies. Similar to an insurance consultant, an 'insurance broker' also shops around for the best insurance policy amongst many companies. However, with insurance brokers, the fee is usually paid in the form of commission from the insurer that is selected rather than directly from the client.

Neither insurance consultants nor insurance brokers are insurance companies and no risks are transferred to them in insurance transactions. Third party administrators are companies that perform underwriting and sometimes claims handling services for insurance companies. These companies often have special expertise that the insurance companies do not have.

Medical/ Health Insurance

Medical/ Health Insurance is an insurance policy where the insurer assures the insured to compensate the loss incurred due to injury or illness. Health insurance offers compensation for medicine, hospitalizations, doctor visit and follows check ups and many other medical expenses. Medical Insurance is often referred to as health insurance and vice versa. Health Insurance can also be done against disability or long term nursing conditions.

The health insurance plans work on a mutual ground, where the insured needs to pay a premium on a regular basis so that the insurer can compensate for any uncertain loss incurred at any point of time.

Medical Insurance are categorized under several plans which differ in various aspect ob the basis of what liabilities they cover, the amount of deductible or co-payments, limits of medical coverage and what all options for treatment the medical policies offers.

Medical Insurance can be done from any private insurer or government insurers. Numerous private insurance companies like the ICICI and Tata AIG to name a few offer medical insurance plans. Health insurance plans can be done as group health plans, individual plans, workers' compensation and government health plans.

Health Insurance Policies in India are sub-divided into the following types of insurance plans:

Hospitalization Plans: this insurance plan assures the insured of covering the hospitalization expense and frequent medical expenses. There is varied pay structure and individual limit as per the plan for the various plans present under this category.

Critical Illness Plans: this insurance plan cover expenses incurred in case of more serious and critical illnesses like heart attack, stroke, organ transplants and kidney failure etc. This medical plan covers infrequent and relatively higher medical expenses.

Specific Conditions Coverage: These medical plans offer health insurance against health complications that might occur due to some disease. These medical plans often include disease management programs related to the condition or the illness.

Health insurance, in today's world is a must for all individual as these insurance policies pay all or part of medical bills.

6.4 TYPES OF INSURANCES

There are four types of insurance: Life, Fire, Marine and Miscellaneous Insurance. Life insurance is treated separately, while Fire, Marine and Miscellaneous insurance all fall within the General Insurance umbrella.

Insurance is mainly protection against future loss. It can be better described as promise of reimbursement in any case of loss. Insurances are paid to people or companies by the insurance company against any kind of hazards or calamities. There are some major types of insurances that include-

- **Health Insurance**
- **Life Insurance**
- **Disability Insurances**
- **Casualty Insurances**
- **Property Insurance**
- **Liability Insurance and**
- **Credit Insurance**

Let's discuss about these major types of insurances along with their features

Health Insurance:

Health insurance policies are offered for any kind of health treatments. This insurance covers all the medical expenses of an individual. It also includes long- term nursing or custodial care needs and disability needs.

- Medical Insurance
- Critical Illness Insurance

Disability Insurances:

This insurance policy provides financial support to the policyholders who are unable to do any kind of work because of their physical disabilities or injuries. It also offers monthly financial support to the policyholders to help them in paying both mortgages and credit cards.

Casualty Insurances:

Casualty Insurances is provided against any kind of accidents and it is categorised as Crime insurance and Political risk insurance.

Life Insurances:

The Insurance Act, 1938, and Insurance Regulatory & Development Authority Act, 1999, have made life insurance in India a federal matter. Therefore, all life insurance companies in India have to comply with the strict regulations laid out by Insurance Regulatory and Development Authority of India (IRDA), irrespective of whether they are state-owned (Life Insurance Corporation of India) or private (ICICI Prudential Life Insurance, Bajaj Allianz Life Insurance Company).

Life Insurances are such kind of insurances that are paid to named beneficiaries when the insured person dies. Life insurance provides a monetary benefit to the family member or a relative to a decedent. It also includes several policies that include-

Endowment Policy

Whole Life Insurance Policy

Money Back Policy

Joint Life Insurance Policy

Group Insurance

Term Life Insurance Policy

Pension Plan

Property Insurance:

In this insurance, an insurance holder can get protection against any kind of risks to property including theft or natural calamities. Property insurance also includes-

Fire Insurance

Flood insurance

Home Insurance

Earthquake Insurance

Inland marine Insurance or Boiler Insurance.

Automobile Insurance

Aviation Insurance

Builder's Risk Insurance

Crop Insurance

Terrorism Insurance

Volcano Insurance

Windstorm Insurance, etc.

Apart from these categories, there are several general insurance categories that include-

Medical/ Health Insurance

Travel Insurance

Auto Insurance

Agricultural Insurance

Commercial Insurance and many others.

Dental Insurance

Dental insurance covers dental costs for an individual or group. The costs include normal dental care cost as well as damage to teeth in an accident. Dental insurance protects people from financial hardship caused by unexpected dental expenses.

Automobile insurance

Auto insurance protects the policy owner against financial loss if he has an accident. It is a contract between policy owner and the insurance company. The policy owner agrees to pay the premium and the insurance company agrees to pay the losses as defined in your policy.

- Two Wheeler Insurance
- Car Insurance
- Commercial Vehicle Insurance

Property insurance

Property insurance gives protection against your property. This includes specialized forms of insurance like fire insurance, flood insurance, earthquake insurance, home insurance etc.

Property insurance provides protection against risks to property, such as fire, theft or weather damage. This includes specialized forms of insurance such as fire insurance, flood insurance, earthquake insurance, home insurance, inland marine insurance or boiler insurance.

- *Automobile insurance*, known in the UK as *motor insurance*, is probably the most common form of insurance and may cover both legal liability claims against the driver and loss of or damage to the insured's vehicle itself. Throughout the United States an auto insurance policy is required to legally operate a motor vehicle on public roads. In some jurisdictions, bodily injury compensation for automobile accident victims has been changed to a no-fault system, which reduces or eliminates the ability to sue for compensation but provides automatic eligibility for benefits. Credit card companies insure against damage on rented cars.

    o   Driving School Insurance insurance provides cover for any authorized driver whilst undergoing tuition, cover also unlike other motor policies provides cover for instructor liability where both the pupil and driving instructor are equally liable in the event of a claim.

- *Aviation insurance* insures against hull, spares, deductibles, hull wear and liability risks.

- *Boiler insurance* (also known as boiler and machinery insurance or equipment breakdown insurance) insures against accidental physical damage to equipment or machinery.

- *Builder's risk insurance* insures against the risk of physical loss or damage to property during construction. Builder's risk insurance is typically written on an "all risk" basis covering damage due to any cause (including the negligence of the insured) not otherwise expressly excluded.

- *Crop insurance:* "Farmers use crop insurance to reduce or manage various risks associated with growing crops. Such risks include crop loss or damage caused by weather, hail, drought, frost damage, insects, or disease, for instance."[11]

- *Earthquake insurance* is a form of property insurance that pays the policyholder in the event of an earthquake that causes damage to the property. Most ordinary homeowners insurance policies do not cover earthquake damage. Most earthquake insurance policies feature a high deductible. Rates depend on location and the probability of an earthquake, as well as the construction of the home.

- A *fidelity bond* is a form of casualty insurance that covers policyholders for losses that they incur as a result of fraudulent acts by specified individuals. It usually insures a business for losses caused by the dishonest acts of its employees.

- *Flood insurance* protects against property loss due to flooding. Many insurers in the U.S. do not provide flood insurance in some portions of the country. In response to this, the federal government created the National Flood Insurance Program which serves as the insurer of last resort.

- *Landlord insurance* is specifically designed for people who own properties which they rent out. Most house insurance cover in the U.K will not be valid if the property is rented out therefore landlords must take out this specialist form of home insurance.

- *Marine insurance* and *marine cargo insurance* cover the loss or damage of ships at sea or on inland waterways, and of the cargo that may be on them. When the owner of the cargo and the carrier are separate corporations, marine cargo insurance typically compensates the owner of cargo for losses sustained from fire, shipwreck, etc., but excludes losses that can be recovered from the carrier or the carrier's insurance. Many marine insurance underwriters will include "time element" coverage in such policies, which extends the indemnity to cover loss of profit and other business expenses attributable to the delay caused by a covered loss.

- *Surety bond insurance* is a three party insurance guaranteeing the performance of the principal.

- *Terrorism insurance* provides protection against any loss or damage caused by terrorist activities.

- *Volcano insurance* is an insurance that covers volcano damage in Hawaii.

- *Windstorm insurance* is an insurance covering the damage that can be caused by hurricanes and tropical cyclones.

Travel Insurance

The insurance sector over a period of time has developed into a well organised sector where participation from the public sector and private insurance companies have resulted in a large number of insurance seekers. Insurance is a serious business in India and both the private and public sector participation has further scaled up the need for insurance in India.

Agriculture Insurance

India is an agrarian society with 75% of the population depending on it, for their livelihood. Agriculture or crop insurance has assumed importance with large scale damage caused due to pest attacks, crop diseases and vagaries of weather. The objective is to provide insurance coverage and financial support to the farmers in the event of failure of any of the notified crop as a result of natural calamities, pests & diseases. The list of crops being covered for insurance differs from state to state. Generally quite a few Kharif and Rabi season crops are covered. These crops are insured at the community/block/gram panchayat levels. Agriculture insurance schemes are of immense help to farmers, providing them with financial security.

Fire Insurance

Fire Insurance is governed by All India Fire Tariff effective from 31.3.2001 issued by Tariff Advisory Committee, a Statutory Body. It is a commercial policy covering building, offices, machinery, contents and personal belongings of the office. It mitigates the risk of loss of customers arising from fire breakout. The insured should take all possible steps to minimize the loss.

Term Insurance

Term insurance covers you for a term of one or more years. It pays a death benefit only if the policy holder dies during the period the insurance is in force. Term insurance generally offers the cheapest form of life insurance. You can renew most term insurance policies for one or more terms even if your health condition has changed.

However, each time you renew the policy for a new term, premiums may climb higher, just like a rent agreement every time you renew the lease. This policy is particularly useful to cover any outstanding debt in the form of a mortgage, home loan, etc.

For example if you have taken a loan of Rs10 lakh, you will have an option of taking an insurance to protect the loan in case of passing away before the debt is repaid.

Whole Life Insurance

Whole life insurance covers you for as long as you live if your premiums are paid. You generally pay the same premium amount throughout your lifetime.

Some whole life policies let you pay premiums for a shorter period such as 15, 20 or 25 years. Premiums for these policies are higher since the premium payments are made during a shorter period. There are options in the market to have a return of premium option in a whole life policy. That means after a certain age of paying premiums, the life insurance company will pay back the premium to the life assured but the coverage will continue.

Money Back Insurance

The money back plan not only covers your life, it also assures you the return of a certain per cent of the sum assured as cash payment at regular intervals. It is a savings plan with the added advantage of life cover and regular cash inflow. This plan is ideal for planning special moments like a wedding, your child's education or purchase of an asset, etc. Money back plan have "participating" and "non participating" versions in the market.

Endowment Assurance

Endowment insurance is a level premium plan with a savings feature. At maturity, a lump sum is paid out equal to the sum assured (plus dividends in a par policy). If death occurs during the term of the policy then the total amount of insurance and any dividends (par policy) are paid out.

There are a number of products in the market that offer flexibility in choosing the term of the policy namely you can choose the term from five to 30 years. There are products in the market that offer non participating (no profits) version, the premiums for which are cheaper

Universal Life

This is a flexible life insurance policy and is also market sensitive. You decide on the several investment options on how your net premium are to be invested. While the mony invested has the potential for significant growth, such funds are subject to market risks including the loss of the principal.

Unit Linked Product

Market-linked plans or unit-linked insurance plans (ULIP) are similar to traditional insurance policies with the exception that your premium amount is invested by the insurance company in the stock market.

Market-linked insurance plans (MLP) mimic mutual funds and invest in a basket of securities, allowing you to choose between investment options predominantly in equity, debt or a mix of both (called balanced option).

The major advantage market-linked plans offer is that they leave the asset allocation decision in the hands of investors themselves. You are in control of how you want to distribute your money among the broad class of instruments and when you want to do it or pull out. Any of the products mentioned above except term products could be unit-linked.

Riders

Riders are additional add-on benefits that you could opt to include in your policy over and above what the policy may provide. However, these additions come at an extra premium charge depending of the rider you opt for. These riders cannot be bought separately and independently. The extra premium, nature and characteristics of the riders are based on the base policy that is offered.

Some riders available in the market are :

- *Accident Death Benefit:* Provides a additional amount in case death occurs as a result of an accident.
- *Term Rider:* It allows the payment of an additional amount should death of the insured happens.
- *Waiver of Premium:* In case of total and permanent disability of life insured due to accident or any other means this rider allows premiums on base policy or riders to be waived.
- *Critical Illness:* It provides payment of an additional amount on the diagnosis of some critical illness.

Commercial Insurance Claim Procedure:

The insurer needs to submit all the original documents of the commercial in the case of any financial or non financial loss. The surveyor calculates the approximate value of the loss so incurred. Based on the report submitted by the surveyor, insurance companies pay the amount of loss incurred. The claims are generally cleared within 7-21 days.

Documents Required for Commercial Insurance Claim:

1. Claim Form
2. List of things or items lost or damaged
3. Proof of ownership of business

List of Some of Insurance Companies Offering Commercial/ Business Insurance:

- **Bajaj Allianz** - Corporate Insurance
- **ICICI Lombard** - Business Products
- **United India Insurance Co.** - Business Policies
- **The New India Assurance Co.** - Commercial Products

6.5 TYPES OF INSURANCE POLICIES

Insurance provides compensation to a person for an anticipated loss to his life, business or an asset. Insurance is broadly classified into two parts covering different types of risks:

1. Long-term (Life Insurance)

2. General Insurance (Non-life Insurance)

Long-term Insurance

Long term insurance is so called because it is meant for a long-term period which may stretch to several years or whole life-time of the insured. Long-term insurance covers all policies. Insurance against risk to one's life is covered under ordinary life assurance. Ordinary life assurance can be further classified into following types.

Types of Ordinary Life Assurance Meaning

1. **Whole Life Assurance** : In whole life assurance, insurance company collects premium from the insured for whole life or till the time of his retirement and pays claim to the family of the insured only after his death.

2. **Endowment Assurance:** In case of endowment assurance, the term of policy is defined for a specified period say 15, 20, 25 or 30 years. The insurance company pays the claim to the family of assured in an event of his death within the policy's term or in an event of the assured surviving the policy's term.

3. **Assurances for Children:**

   i) Child's Deferred Assurance: Under this policy, claim by insurance company is paid on the option date which is calculated to coincide with the child's eighteenth or twenty first birthday. In case the parent survives till option date, policy may either be continued or payment may be claimed on the same date. However, if the parent dies before the option date, the policy remains continued until the option date without any need for payment of premiums. If the child dies before the option date, the parent receives back all premiums paid to the insurance company.

   ii) School fee policy: School fee policy can be availed by effecting an endowment policy, on the life of the parent with the sum assured, payable in instalments over the schooling period.

4. **Term Assurance:** The basic feature of term assurance plans is that they provide death risk-cover. Term assurance policies are only for a limited time, claim for which is paid to the family of the assured only when he dies. In case the assured survives the term of policy, no claim is paid to the assured.

5. **Annuities:** Annuities are just opposite to life insurance. A person entering into an annuity contract agrees to pay a specified sum of capital (lump sum or by instalments) to the insurer. The insurer in return promises to pay the insured a series of payments untill insured's death. Generally, life annuity is opted by a person having surplus wealth and wants to use this money after his retirement.There are two types of annuities, namely:Immediate Annuity: In an immediate annuity, the insured pays a lump sum amount (known as purchase price) and in return the insurer promises to pay him in instalments a specified sum on a monthly/quarterly/half-yearly/yearly basis. Deferred Annuity: A deferred anuuity can be purchased by paying a single premium or by way of instalments. The insured starts receiving annuity payment after a lapse of a selected period (also known as Deferment period).

6. **Money Back Policy:** Money back policy is a policy opted by people who want periodical payments. A money back policy is generally issued for a particular period, and the sum assured is paid through periodical payments to the insured, spread over this time period. In case of death of the insured within the term of the policy, full sum assured along with bonus accruing on it is payable by hte insurance company to the nominee of the deceased.

6.6 GENERAL INSURANCE

Also known as non-life insurance, general insurance is normally meant for a short-term period of twelve months or less. Recently, longer-term insurance agreements have made an entry into the business of general insurance but their term does not exceed five years. General insurance can be classified as follows:

Fire Insurance: Fire insurance provides protection against damage to property caused by accidents due to fire, lightening or explosion, whereby the explosion is caused by boilers not being used for industrial purposes. Fire insurance also includes damage caused due to other perils like strom tempest or flood; burst pipes; earthquake; aircraft; riot, civil commotion; malicious damage; explosion; impact.

Marine Insurance: Marine insurance basically covers three risk areas, namely, hull, cargo and freight. The risks which these areas are exposed to are collectively known as "Perils of the Sea". These perils include theft, fire, collision etc.

Marine Cargo: Marine cargo policy provides protection to the goods loaded on a ship against all perils between the departure and arrival warehouse. Therefore, marine cargo covers carriage of goods by sea as well as transportation of goods by land.

Marine Hull: Marine hull policy provides protection against damage to ship caused due to the perils of the sea. Marine hull policy covers three-fourth of the liability of the hull owner (shipowner) against loss due to collisions at sea. The remaining 1/4th of the liability is looked after by associations formed by shipowners for the purpose (P and I clubs).

Miscellaneous As per the Insurance Act, all types of general insurance other than fire and marine insurance are covered under miscellaneous insurance. Some of the examples of general insurance are motor insurance, theft insurance, health insurance, personal accident insurance, money insurance, engineering insurance etc.

6.7 MARINE INSURANCE

Marine insurance falls under commercial insurance. The policy is taken to reduce business risks. It caters to small scale business organisations to large corporates. Policy does not cover loss or damage due to willful misconduct, ordinary leakage, improper packing, delay, war, strike, riot and civil commotion.

Marine Insurance covers the loss or damage of ships, cargo, terminals, and any transport or property by which cargo is transferred, acquired, or held between the points of origin and final destination. Cargo insurance—discussed here—is a sub-branch of marine insurance, though Marine also includes Onshore and Offshore exposed property (container terminals, ports, oil platforms, pipelines); Hull; Marine Casualty; and Marine Liability.

Different types of Marine Insurance are available:

*   Marine import transit insurance
*   Marine export transit insurance
*   Marine inland transit insurance
*   Marine insurance claim procedure
*   Marine Hull

Calculation of Marine Insurance Amount/Premium:

Amount of premium depends on factors like nature of cargo, scope of cover, packing, mode of conveyance, distance and past claims experience. Premium can be paid on a monthly/quarterly/half-yearly/yearly basis.

Marine Insurance Claim Procedure:

*   In case of loss/damage in transit, a monetary claim should be lodged with the carrier within the time limit to protect recovery rights
*   Appointment of surveyor or claim representative in agreement with the insurer to determine the nature, cause and extent of loss/damage
*   The surveyor informs the insurer of the approximate value of loss incurred
*   The claim procedure takes from one to three weeks

Origins of Formal Marine Insurance

The modern origins of marine insurance law were in the law merchant, with the establishment in England in 1601 of a specialised chamber of assurance separate from the other Courts. Lord Mansfield, Lord Chief Justice in the mid-eighteenth century, began the merging of law merchant and common law principles. The establishment of Lloyd's of London, competitor insurance companies, a developing infrastructure of specialists (such as shipbrokers, admiralty lawyers, and bankers), and the growth of the British Empire gave English law a prominence in this area which it largely maintains and forms the basis of almost all modern practice. The growth of the London insurance market led to the standardisation of policies and judicial precedent further developed marine insurance law. In 1906 the Marine Insurance Act was passed which codified the previous common law; it is both an extremely thorough and concise piece of work. Although the title of the Act refers to marine insurance, the general principles have been applied to all non-life insurance.

- In the 19th. century, Lloyd's and the Institute of London Underwriters (a grouping of London company insurers) developed between them standardised clauses for the use of marine insurance, and these have been maintained since. These are known as the Institute Clauses because the Institute covered the cost of their publication.

- Within the overall guidance of the Marine Insurance Act and the Institute Clauses parties retain a considerable freedom to contract between themselves.

- Marine insurance is the oldest type of insurance. Out of it grew non-marine insurance and reinsurance. It traditionally formed the majority of business underwritten at Lloyd's. Nowadays, Marine insurance is often grouped with Aviation and Transit (ie. cargo) risks, and in this form is known by the acronym 'MAT'

Different types of Marine Insurance are available:

- Marine import transit insurance
- Marine export transit insurance
- Marine inland transit insurance
- Marine insurance claim procedure
- Marine Hull

Calculation of Marine Insurance Amount/Premium:

Amount of premium depends on factors like nature of cargo, scope of cover, packing, mode of conveyance, distance and past claims experience. Premium can be paid on a monthly/quarterly/half-yearly/yearly basis.

Marine Insurance Claim Procedure:

- In case of loss/damage in transit, a monetary claim should be lodged with the carrier within the time limit to protect recovery rights
- Appointment of surveyor or claim representative in agreement with the insurer to determine the nature, cause and extent of loss/damage
- The surveyor informs the insurer of the approximate value of loss incurred
- The claim procedure takes from one to three weeks

Documents Required for Marine Insurance Claim:

1. Original Invoice & packing List - if forming part of Invoice
2. Document of declaration of consignment
3. Damage Certificate from the carrier

Organizations offering Marine Insurance:

- ICICI Lombard - Marine Import Transit Insurance Policy
- United India Insurance Co. - Marine Cargo
- The New India Assurance Co. - Marine Cargo Policy

6.8 HEALTH INSURANCE

Health care costs have witnessed a phenomenal rise in the current times, this has led the customers to insure not only themselves but their family members for any future medical expenses and other related requirements. The need to insure assumes even more importance with older generation who are either retired or will be retired in the near future; you will be surprised how much health care expenses can add up to in a year.

Health insurance is <u>insurance</u> that pays for medical expenses. It is sometimes used more broadly to include insurance covering <u>disability</u> or <u>long-term nursing or custodial care</u> needs. It may be provided through a government-sponsored <u>social insurance</u> program, or from private insurance companies. It may be purchased on a group basis (e.g., by a firm to cover its employees) or purchased by individual consumers. In each case, the covered groups or individuals pay premiums or taxes to help protect themselves from high or unexpected healthcare expenses. Similar benefits paying for medical expenses may also be provided through social welfare programs funded by the government.

By estimating the overall risk of healthcare expenses, a routine finance structure (such as a monthly premium or annual tax) can be developed, ensuring that money is available to pay for the healthcare benefits specified in the insurance agreement. The benefit is administered by a central organization such as a government agency, private business, or not-for-profit entity.

History and evolution

The concept of health insurance was proposed in 1694 by Hugh the Elder Chamberlen from the Peter Chamberlen family. In the late 19th century, "accident insurance" began to be available, which operated much like modern *disability* insurance. This payment model continued until the start of the 20th century in some jurisdictions (like California), where all laws regulating health insurance actually referred to disability insurance.

Accident insurance was first offered in the United States by the Franklin Health Assurance Company of Massachusetts. This firm, founded in 1850, offered insurance against injuries arising from railroad and steamboat accidents. Sixty organizations were offering accident insurance in the U.S. by 1866, but the industry consolidated rapidly soon thereafter. While there were earlier experiments, the origins of sickness coverage in the U.S. effectively date from 1890. The first employer-sponsored group disability policy was issued in 1911.

Before the development of medical expense insurance, patients were expected to pay all other health care costs out of their own pockets, under what is known as the fee-for-service business model. During the middle to late 20th century, traditional disability insurance evolved into modern health insurance programs. Today, most comprehensive private health insurance programs cover the cost of routine, preventive, and emergency health care procedures, and also most prescription drugs, but this was not always the case.

Hospital and medical expense policies were introduced during the first half of the 20th century. During the 1920s, individual hospitals began offering services to individuals on a pre-paid basis, eventually leading to the development of Blue Cross organizations. The predecessors of today's Health Maintenance Organizations (HMOs) originated beginning in 1929, through the 1930s and on during World War II

A health insurance policy is a contract between an insurance company and an individual or his sponsor (e.g. an employer). The contract can be renewable annually or monthly. The type and amount of health care costs that will be covered by the health insurance company are specified in advance, in the member contract or "Evidence of Coverage" booklet. The individual insurered person's obligations may take several forms:

- **Premium:** The amount the policy-holder or his sponsor (e.g. an employer) pays to the health plan each month to purchase health coverage.

- **Deductible:** The amount that the insured must pay out-of-pocket before the health insurer pays its share. For example, a policy-holder might have to pay a $500 deductible per year, before any of their health care is covered by the health insurer. It may take several doctor's visits or prescription refills before the insured person reaches the deductible and the insurance company starts to pay for care.

- **Copayment:** The amount that the insured person must pay out of pocket before the health insurer pays for a particular visit or service. For example, an insured person might pay a $45 copayment for a doctor's visit, or to obtain a prescription. A copayment must be paid each time a particular service is obtained.

- **Coinsurance:** Instead of, or in addition to, paying a fixed amount up front (a copayment), the co-insurance is a percentage of the total cost that insured person may also pay. For example, the member might have to pay 20% of the cost of a surgery over and above a co-payment, while the insurance company pays the other 80%. If there is an upper limit on coinsurance, the policy-holder could end up owing very little, or a great deal, depending on the actual costs of the services they obtain.

- **Exclusions:** Not all services are covered. The insured person is generally expected to pay the full cost of non-covered services out of their own pocket.

- **Coverage limits:** Some health insurance policies only pay for health care up to a certain dollar amount. The insured person may be expected to pay any charges in excess of the health plan's maximum payment for a specific service. In addition, some insurance company schemes have annual or lifetime coverage maximums. In these cases, the health plan will stop payment when they reach the benefit maximum, and the policy-holder must pay all remaining costs.

- **Out-of-pocket maximums:** Similar to coverage limits, except that in this case, the insured person's payment obligation ends when they reach the out-of-pocket maximum, and the health company pays all further covered costs. Out-of-pocket maximums can be limited to a specific benefit category (such as prescription drugs) or can apply to all coverage provided during a specific benefit year.

- **Capitation:** An amount paid by an insurer to a health care provider, for which the provider agrees to treat all members of the insurer.

- **In-Network Provider:** (U.S. term) A health care provider on a list of providers preselected by the insurer. The insurer will offer discounted coinsurance or copayments, or additional benefits, to a plan member to see an in-network provider. Generally, providers in network are providers who have a contract with the insurer to accept rates further discounted from the "usual and customary" charges the insurer pays to out-of-network providers.

- **Prior Authorization:** A certification or authorization that an insurer provides prior to medical service occurring. Obtaining an authorization means that the insurer is obligated to pay for the service, assume it matches what was authorized. Many smaller, routine services do not require authorization.

- **Explanation of Benefits:** A document sent by an insurer to a patient explaining what was covered for a medical service, and how they arrived at the payment amount and patient responsibility amount.

6.9 INSURANCE SECTOR IN INDIA

The insurance sector in India has come a full circle from being an open competitive market to nationalisation and back to a liberalised market again. Tracing the developments in the Indian insurance sector reveals the 360-degree turn witnessed over a period of almost two centuries.

A brief history of the Insurance sector

The business of life insurance in India in its existing form started in India in the year 1818 with the establishment of the Oriental Life Insurance Company in Calcutta.

Some of the important milestones in the life insurance business in India are:

- 1912: The Indian Life Assurance Companies Act enacted as the first statute to regulate the life insurance business.

- 1928: The Indian Insurance Companies Act enacted to enable the government to collect statistical information about both life and non-life insurance businesses.

- 1938: Earlier legislation consolidated and amended to by the Insurance Act with the objective of protecting the interests of the insuring public.

- 1956: 245 Indian and foreign insurers and provident societies taken over by the central government and nationalised. LIC formed by an Act of Parliament, viz. LIC Act, 1956, with a capital contribution of Rs. 5 crore from the Government of India.

The General insurance business in India, on the other hand, can trace its roots to the Triton Insurance Company Ltd., the first general insurance company established in the year 1850 in Calcutta by the British.

Some of the important milestones in the general insurance business in India are:

- 1907: The Indian Mercantile Insurance Ltd. set up, the first company to transact all classes of general insurance business.

- 1957: General Insurance Council, a wing of the Insurance Association of India, frames a code of conduct for ensuring fair conduct and sound business practices.

- 1968: The Insurance Act amended to regulate investments and set minimum solvency margins and the Tariff Advisory Committee set up.

- 1972: The General Insurance Business (Nationalisation) Act, 1972 nationalised the general insurance business in India with effect from 1st January 1973.

- 107 insurers amalgamated and grouped into four companies viz. the National Insurance Company Ltd., the New India Assurance Company Ltd., the Oriental Insurance Company Ltd. and the United India Insurance Company Ltd. GIC incorporated as a company.

Insurance sector reforms:

In 1993, Malhotra Committee headed by former Finance Secretary and RBI Governor R.N. Malhotra was formed to evaluate the Indian insurance industry and recommend its future direction.

The Malhotra committee was set up with the objective of complementing the reforms initiated in the financial sector. The reforms were aimed at "creating a more efficient and competitive financial system suitable for the requirements of the economy keeping in mind the structural changes currently underway and recognizing that insurance is an important part of the overall financial system where it was necessary to address the need for similar reforms

6.10 TYPES OF HEALTH CARE INSURANCE AVAILABLE:

Medical Insurance

Medical insurance in India is gaining such a high trend that policies are out even for infants. It is the buffer against medical emergencies. This cover is a hospitalisation cover and reimbursement of the medical expenses incurred in respect of covered disease /surgery while the insured was admitted in the hospital as an in patient.

Different types of Medical Insurance are available here:

- Individual Medical Insurance
- Group Medical Insurance
- Overseas Medical Insurance

Calculation of Medical Insurance Amount/Premium:

The amount of premium depends on the sum insured (amount of coverage) age of the member and also if one is taking an individual or a group Insurance. Premium can be paid on a monthly/quarterly/half yearly/ yearly basis. Amount also depends on the company policies of the insured.

Medical Insurance Claim Procedure:

- An individual has to fill and submit the claim form to the insurer
- A claim representative, so appointed, analyses the expenses incurred
- After submission of the medical expenses report, the claim is cleared within 7-15 days. The number of days may vary from company to company

Documents Required for Medical Insurance Claim:

- Hospital/doctor report
- Memo of expenses incurred
- Salary Slip

List of Common Insurance Companies Offering Medical Insurance:

- **United India Insurance Co.** - Mediclaim Policy
- **The New India Assurance Co.** - Medical Plans
- **ICICI Loambard** - Online Medical Plans
- **Bajaj Allianz** - Medical Care
- **HSBC** - HealthFirst

Critical Illness Insurance

Critical Illness Insurance provides for payment of amount equal to sum assured, if illness strikes, irrespective of expenses incurred on treatment. Most insurance companies are providing this insurance as an addition to the life insurance; additional premium payable for critical illness. It is introduced as a value addition to meet the demands and also as marketing strategy. The insurance covers surgery cost, critical illness cover and post-hospitalisation. The insurance is different in paying only for prolonged hospitalisations. One of the unique features of this insurance is that a lump sum allowance is paid irrespective of the actual medical expenses.

Calculation of Critical Illness Insurance Amount/Premium:

The amount of premium depends on the insurance of the insurance company. Sometimes life insurance companies charge extra premium for the insurance, which is an add on to the LIP. Premium is generally paid on a yearly basis.

Critical Illness Insurance Claim Procedure:

Insurance holders can make multiple claims till their lifetime cover is exhausted. The company pays a lumpsum amount as claims irrespective of the actual expenses, as against a medical insurance, which is only a reimbursement insurance. The claim should be reported to the insurers, who in turn will appoint a surveyor. Surveyor will check the necessary documents and analyse the extent of damage. The claim process takes anywhere from 7-21 days.

Documents Required for Critical Illness Insurance Claim:

1. Copy of FIR (If any)

2. Medical Certificate & details of medical expenses & disability certificate

3. Leave certificate from employer

4. Duly filled Claim Form

5. Salary Certificate from employer

List of Some of Insurance Companies Offering Critical Illness Insurance:

- **Bajaj Allianz** - Insurance Against Serious Illness
- **HSBC** - Illness Cover
- **Life Insurance Co.** - Critical Illness Benefit Rider

SUMMARY

In India there are about 250 large pharmaceutical manufacturers and about 8000 small scale pharmaceutical manufacturers. The total worth of Pharmaceutical industries is said to be about around $ 4 million and it is said to be growing at a rate of 10 to 12% annually. Insurance is a mean to remove the hindrance of risk. There are life insurance, fire insurance, marine insurance, car insurance, medical insurance and many more insurance facilities given by insurance companies

There are four types of insurance: Life, Fire, Marine and Miscellaneous Insurance. Life insurance is treated separately, while Fire, Marine and Miscellaneous insurance all fall within the General Insurance umbrella.

Medical/ Health Insurance is an insurance policy where the insurer assures the insured to compensate the loss incurred due to injury or illness. Health insurance offers compensation for medicine, hospitalizations, doctor visit and follows check ups and many other medical expenses. Medical Insurance is often referred to as health insurance and vice versa.

Marine insurance falls under commercial insurance. The policy is taken to reduce business risks. It caters to small scale business organizations to large corporates. Policy does not cover loss or damage due to willful misconduct, ordinary leakage, improper packing, delay, war, strike, riot and civil commotion. Marine

Insurance covers the loss or damage of ships, cargo, terminals, and any transport or property by which cargo is transferred, acquired, or held between the points of origin and final destination. Cargo insurance—discussed here—is a sub-branch of marine insurance, though Marine also includes Onshore and Offshore exposed property (container terminals, ports, oil platforms, pipelines); Hull; Marine Casualty; and Marine Liability.

REVIEW QUESTIONS

1. Explain briefly the insurance scenario in India?

2. What are the different types of insurances meet the different purposes of risk?

3. What is life insurance and explain the relationships between the insurer and insured?

4. Write brief note on the property insurance and explain how it is useful to the pharmaceutical store?

5. What is general insurance? Discuss the various general insurance policies available to the customers

6. Discuss in detail the intricacies involved in marine insurance?

7. Explain the various types of marine insurances?

8. Briefly discuss the insurance industry over the years since independences?

9. Explain the concept of health insurance and discuss the merits and demerits in it?

10. Enumerate the different insurance companies working India under private and public ownerships?

Chapter 7

GOVERNANCE IN PHARMACY

7. 1 INTRODUCTION TO PHARMACY COUNCILS

Governance in pharmacy means to understand the associations, societies an statutory councils which monitor, regulate and control the functioning and performance of the pharmaceutical companies.

Pharmacy Council of India (PCI)

The Pharmacy education and profession in India up to graduate level is regulated by the PCI, a statutory body governed by the provisions of the Pharmacy Act, 1948 passed by the Parliament.

The Pharmacy Act 1948 was enacted on 4.3.1948 with the following preamble- "An Act to regulate the profession of pharmacy. Whereas it is expedient to make better provision for the regulation of the profession and practice of pharmacy and for that purpose to constitute Pharmacy Councils".

Objectives of PCI

The PCI was constituted on 9.8.1949 under section 3 of the Pharmacy Act with following objectives:

- Regulation of the Pharmacy Education in the Country for the purpose of registration as a pharmacist under the Pharmacy Act.
- Regulation of Profession and Practice of Pharmacy.

Constitution and composition of central council

The Central Government shall, as soon as may be, constitute a Central Council consisting of the following members, namely: -

(a) Six members, among whom there shall be at least one teacher of each of the subjects, pharmaceutical chemistry, pharmacy, pharmacology and pharmacognosy elected by the [University Grants Commission] from among persons on the teaching staff of an Indian University or a college affiliated thereto which grants a degree or diploma in pharmacy.

(b)   six members, of whom at least [four] shall be persons possessing a degree or diploma in, and practicing pharmacy or pharmaceutical chemistry, nominated by the Central Government.

(c)   One member elected from amongst themselves by the members of the Medical Council of India;

(d)   The Director General, Health Services, *ex officio* or if he is unable to attend any meeting, a person authorized by him in writing to do so.

[(dd)] the Drugs Controller, India, *ex officio* or if he is unable to attend any meeting, a person authorised by him in writing to do so.

(e)   The Director of the Central Drugs Laboratory, *ex officio*.

(f)   a representative of the University Grants Commission and a representative of the All India Council for Technical Education.

(g)   one member to represent each State elected [from amongst themselves] by the members of each State Council, who shall be a registered pharmacist.

(h)   one member to represent each State nominated by [the] State Government, who shall be a registered pharmacist.

7.2   CONSTITUTION AND COMPOSITION OF STATE COUNCILS.

The State Government shall constitute a State Council consisting of the following members, namely:

(a)   six members, elected from amongst themselves by registered pharmacists of the State.

(b)   five members, of whom at least [three] shall be persons possessing a prescribed degree or diploma in pharmacy or pharmaceutical chemistry or [registered pharmacists], nominated by the State Government.

(c)   One member elected from amongst themselves by the members of each Medical Council or the Council of Medical Registration of the State, as the case may be.

(d)   the chief administrative medical officer of the State *ex officio* or if he is unable to attend any meeting, a person authorized by him in writing to do so.

[(dd)] the officer-in-charge of drugs control organization of the State under the [Drugs and Cosmetics Act, 1940 (23 of 1940)], *ex officio* or if he is unable to attend any meeting, a person authorized by him in writing to do so.

(e) the Government Analyst under the [Drugs and Cosmetics Act, 1940 (23 of 1940)], *ex officio*, or where there is more than one, such one as the State Government may appoint in this behalf.

FUNCTIONS AND DUTIES OF THE COUNCIL

1. To prescribe minimum standard of education required for qualifying as a pharmacist.

2. Framing of Education Regulations prescribing the conditions to be fulfilled by the institutions seeking approval of the PCI for imparting education in pharmacy.

3. To ensure uniform implementation of the educational standards through out the country. Inspection of Pharmacy Institutions seeking approval under the Pharmacy Act to verify availability of the prescribed norms.

4. To approve the course of study and examination for pharmacists i.e. approval of the academic training institutions providing pharmacy courses.

5. To withdraw approval, if the approved course of study or an approved examination does not continue to be in conformity with the educational standards prescribed by the PCI.

6. To approve qualifications granted outside the territories to which the Pharmacy Act extends i.e. the approval of foreign qualification.

7. To maintain Central Register of Pharmacists.

DECISION MAKING PROCEDURE

1. PCI grants approval to a pharmacy institution for the conduct of "Course of Study" and "Examination" for the purpose of registration as a pharmacist.

2. Whenever any prospective institution applies, procedure for seeking approval is intimated.

3. On receipt of duly filled in application and complete documents, an inspection is arranged to verify the availability of prescribed norms.

4. Inspection Report on receipt is forwarded to institution for rectification of the shortcomings, if any, within a stipulated time period.

5. Inspection Report along with the compliance report if received from institution is placed before the Executive Committee of the Council for consideration.

6. The recommendations of the Executive Committee are placed before the Central Council for approval.

7. The decision of the Central Council is conveyed to the institution and all concerned like Examining Authority, State Pharmacy Council etc.

8. Decision regarding approval and withdrawal is also notified in the Gazette of India.

7.3 PHARMACEUTICALS EXPORT PROMOTION COUNCIL (PHARMEXCIL)

The dynamic growth of Indian Pharma Industry, a knowledge based industry, and the recommendations of four major Pharma associations made the Ministry of Commerce & Industry to realize the need for separate export promotion council. Accordingly, Pharmaceuticals Export Promotion Council (PHARMEXCIL) has been set up on 12.5.2004. With its notification No.61 date. 16.3.2005, Director General of Foreign Trade made Pharmexcil the sole agency to issue RCMCs to all Pharma exporters.

The activities of the Council are administered by Committee of Administration consisting of representatives from major Pharma industries in India like J B Chemicals & Pharmaceuticals Limited, Suven Life Sciences Limited, Dr. Reddy's Laboratories, Aurobindo Phrma, Luipin, Ranbaxy, Novarties, Avantis, Ipca, Shasun, Sun Phrma, Zydus Cadila, Glowchem, Calyx etc., apart from Govt. officials from Central govt. and Govt. of Andhra Pradesh. Administrative support to the Council is extended by very rich experienced personnel from various fields like Govt. of India and Pharma industry.

The Role of Council:

Issue of RCMC Organizing Trade delegations/Buyer-Seller Meetings at abroad Organizing Reverse Buyer-Seller Meetings in India Assisting members to get their MDA/ MAI claims refunded from Govt. of India Issue of Certificate of Origin Organizing periodical Seminars/Interactive meetings on exports related issues Make suggestions to Govt. of India on policy issues relating to Pharma exports and Make representations to Govt. of India and other agencies in India and abroad to get amicable solutions for the common problems of the industry.

Categories under Pharmexcil:

Various pharmaceutical items like Bulk Drugs and its intermediates, Formulations, herbal, ayurvedic, unani and homeopathic medicines, biotech and biological products, diagnostics, surgicals, neutraceuticals, and pharma industry related services, collaborative research, contract manufacturing, clinical trials and consultancy etc come under the purview of Pharmexcil.

7.4 PHARMACEUTICAL ASSOCIATIONS IN INDIA

Organisation of Pharmaceutical Producers of India (OPPI)

Organisation of Pharmaceutical Producers of India (OPPI) established in 1965, is a premier association of research based international and large pharmaceutical companies in India and is also a scientific and professional body. It caters to the needs of Research based Pharmaceutical Industry thereby creating and sustaining an environment conducive to innovation and growth, simultaneously, facilitating industry and stakeholders partnership through various advisory and consultative processes to achieve the Healthcare objectives of the Nation.

OPPI Members Follow:

- Good Manufacturing Practices (GMP)
- International Code of Pharmaceutical Marketing Practices
- OPPI's position on Intellectual Property Rights (IPR)

OPPI functions mainly on the following areas:

- Continuous dialogue with the stakeholders
- Actively engage in knowledge creation & knowledge sharing with value addition
- Engage in 'Corporate Academia' Interaction

OPPI identifies itself with the country's national healthcare objectives and encourages its members to make substantial contributions to social concerns and actively promotes Corporate Social Responsibility (CSR).

OPPI is an active member of International Federation of Pharmaceutical Manufacturers Associations (IFPMA), Geneva.

Objectives of OPPI

- To build on India's existing strengths in manufacturing and Distribution and substantially enhance the beginnings made in R&D in order to become one of the leading players in the global pharmaceuticals market.
- To develop a realization that the degree of success that the Industry attains in these areas will be a direct function of the emphasis given to the development of a sound system of Intellectual Property Rights, Biological Sciences Research (particularly genomics and proteomics), Clinical Research & Development and Innovative Process Chemistry.
- To make India a global sourcing base of high quality pharmaceuticals to international consumers.
- To be one of the major creators of intellectual capital and wealth for the economy.

BULK DRUG MANUFACTURERS ASSOCIATION (INDIA)

The Bulk Drug Manufacturers Association (India) was formed in 1991 with Hyderabad as its Head Quarters. This is an all India body representing all the Bulk Drug Manufacturers of India. The Association works for the consolidation of gains of the industry and serves as a catalyst between the government and the industry on the various issues for the growth of the industry.

Objectives

1. To promote the discussion, on all subjects effecting the Bulk Drug Industry in India, among all members and serve as a common forum for formulating their views on all matters including national, economic, financial, commercial and related policies concerning the growth of the Bulk Drug Industry in the country.

2. To create and encourage mutual help and cooperation among the members.

3. To assist and cooperate, in framing the legislative measures, with State / Central Governments or any such authorities on any matters directly or indirectly effecting the industry, and to represent the collective opinion of the industry in this regard.

4. To diffuse among its members information on all matters effecting the bulk drug industry and to print, publish, issue, circulate such papers, periodicals, books, circulars as may seen conductive to any other objectives of the Association.

5. To encourage the discovery and investigate and make known the nature and merits of inventions, which may seem capable of being used by those engaged in Bulk Drug Industry.

6. To formulate methods for developing indigenous as well as export market for Bulk Drugs manufactured in India.

7. To establish or maintain laboratory for testing the quality standards of Bulk Drugs and other allied products and to establish or maintain Research & Development Centre for development of new drugs/improvement in existing drugs / processes etc., or any Hi-tech Research & Training Center, in the interest of the members of bulk drug industry and the country in general.

INDIAN DRUG MANUFACTURERS' ASSOCIATION (IDMA)

Indian Drug Manufacturers' Association (IDMA) was formed in 1961 to help Indian manufacturers and to protect the interest of the Indian consumer. It has a membership of over 600 wholly-Indian large, medium and small companies.

Activities

Various issues of policy or operational nature relating to the structure and implementation of the Drugs Cosmetics Rules at Central or State level are taken up with the authorities through representations and follow-up meetings. Some of the important issues which have been taken up with the authorities in recent times are:

- Extension of validity of WHO-GMP certificates to five years.
- Six months grace period needed for implementation of overseas pharmacopoeia.
- IDMA's representation on DTAB.
- Decentralisation of work regarding registration for import of drugs
- Delay in testing of drugs.
- License/inspection fees for SSI sector.
- Reduction in 4 years period for treating a drug as 'new' drug.
- Adoption of manufacturer's method of analysis in case of dispute.
- Menace of spurious drugs, etc.

7.5 MEDICAL DETAILING

What is Medical detailing?

Medical detailing is an educational activity by sales representatives–'detailers'–eg, from pharmaceutical companies or manufacturers of medical devices, to provide details or scientific information on a product's potential uses, benefits.

Detailing forms one of the most important tools in pharmaceutical marketing and advertising. Obviously the best measure of whether poor not a salesperson is paying his way is to determine if the actual sales in the area served is affected by his presence. In pharmaceutical marketing this is difficult to assess, for many reasons. First, substantial number of patients usually does not have a prescription filled in the area covered by a given salesperson. Moreover, increasing number of people are using mail order to save money on many prescription drugs. The national retried teacher association reported that in 1980 over 4.5 million prescription were filled in their 9 mail order pharmacies.

As part of medical detailing, a medical chart is a confidential document that contains detailed and comprehensive information on an individual and the care experience related to that person.

Principles of medical detailing

The principles show the way for effective implementation of medical detailing process. Medical detailing has applications in hospitals and pharamaceutical marketing.The follwing are the general principles:

1. Define the problem area
2. understand the problem with clarity
3. Prepare a communication message that should be clear
4. Uderstand the target audience and what they want
5. provide information with clarity in voice and audibility in case of handling visual aid
6. Effective communication,use of senses
7. Time management
8. syncronisation of thought

Objectives:

The objective of medical detailing is reinforcing nutrition information to potential users (doctors)/ existing users, Initiating 'Relationship Building' with contacts/ Increasing 'Share Of Stomach for the category, Appropriate use of detailing aids/scientific inputs provided.

- It is to analyse latest marketing trends activities and providing valuable inputs for fine tuning sales & marketing strategies. Medical detail officer is implementing business strategies, maximizing customer satisfaction and responsible for customer relationship management. He is also responsible for visiting Doctor & Medical institutes, giving presentations about MNCs health, nutrition & baby food products, thereby generating prescription & demand of MNCs products, handling channel sales.

- Advertisement of company's product

- To create and arouse interest in the doctores mind regarding products thus influencing his prescribing habit.

- To emphasize the advantages /benefits and salient features of products and services

- To generate more prescriptions

Academic detailing

In medical detailing, academic detailing is one of the few educational interventions that have consistently demonstrated improved physician performance. Educational outreach methods to improve mental health practices in primary care are in need of much additional research. Improving the detection of mental disorders and underused of mental health treatment may prove to be more difficult than reducing the overuse of unnecessary medications

Medical detailing principles would help "advance health care institution to take up initiatives that provide access to and delivery of equitable, high quality, efficient care and prevention services for people living in the Community who suffer from different diseases.

e-DETAILING

e-detailing is the use of the internet as the medium of communication for pharmaceutical sales detailing to physicians. It is a pharmaceutical or medical device firm-sponsored, internet-based program that informs prescribers about products or diseases using digital technology. Therefore many formats are possible including use of technologies, such as the internet, video-conferencing and interactive voice conferencing for enabling the interaction with the physician.

e-detailing is defined e-detailing as promotion of pharmaceutical products using an online channel and information technology, versus a traditional, off-line channel. Importantly, e-detailing has become more complex than merely just using the internet to detail to physicians.

e-detailing systems vary in interactivity from those that provide relatively static product information online to those that require physicians to go through interactive product materials online and to those that involve the physician in a video conference via the computer. The following is an illustration of the two main types of e-detailing: interactive and video.

e-detailing simply means using digital technology in the **sales detailing process**. **Pharmaceutical companies** use it to communicate product and service messages and related information to healthcare professionals. Doctors in the United States are highly time pressured and encouraged to see as many patients as possible. This means that they often do not have the time to meet with **pharmaceutical sales representatives**. There is no doubt that detailing directly to the doctor serves an important purpose. Doctors want and need information from sales representatives - but on their own time terms. **e-detailing provides** doctors with a more convenient means of getting the information they want at a time that suits them. eDetailing enables the doctor to use a personal computer to launch a sponsored learning application, often consisting of a series of interactive screens with multi-media information about the promoted product, including research evidence, clinical practice guidelines, prescribing information and patient advice. eDetailing is not seen as a replacement to sales representative visits, but rather as a valuable additional channel to receiving information about **pharmaceutical products and services.**

Types of e-detailing
Virtual (interactive) e-detailing

Virtual or interactive e-detailing is a self-service product presentation that physicians can access in their own time. The level of interaction can range from limited product information on handheld devices to more interactive web pages with incentive driven exercises. Interactive websites are the most common form of e-detailing program used by physicians in the USA, France, and the UK. The appeal of such programs is that the physician is in control of its use. During a typical e-detailing program, physicians are presented with a series of interactive learning exercises that reinforce messages specific to a pharmaceutical company's product. At the end of the exercise, physicians are asked whether they would like to receive samples, to meet a sales representative, to participant in market research surveys, or to request literature.

Video (live) e-detailing

Video e-detailing is defined as face-to-face PC-based video conferencing between a physician and a pharmaceutical representative. Usually, physicians in this type of e-detailing are provided with a preconfigured personal computer with all necessary applications preloaded and a webcam to see and speak with a sales representative. The video image of the representative is displayed while audio communication is conducted over the telephone or microphone. Information about product indications, efficacy, dosage, side effects, and clinical data on new and existing products can also appear on the computer screen. In this type of e-detailing, a physician can ask questions via a web interface.

e-detailing process

Pharmaceutical companies that want to inform physicians about drugs or treatment methods via the internet have to abide by certain legal restrictions. Regulations governing pharmaceutical promotion are less restrictive in the USA than in Europe . Many companies control access to their product websites with password protection technology. Pharmaceutical companies allow access to a large number of physicians across different therapy areas. For example, if one pharmaceutical company wants to launch an e-detailing program, then it could contact a vendor and use it to send product information in the form of an email newsletter to a designated physician group. Pharmaceutical companies target physicians through mail, e-mail.. Target physicians will receive an invitation with an invitation number included. Usually, physicians will visit a web site (most of the time a third party vendor company) and use their invitation number to create a personal account with them. Finally, participants can watch interactive presentations, interactive e-detailing, or speak directly with a PSR through, video e-detailing. Certainly, companies introducing a product through the vendor company will target physicians who regularly use the internet and try to raise awareness of its product prior to its launch.

7.6 MAJOR LEGISLATIONS:

There are various legislations that govern the manufacture and sale of drugs and pharmaceuticals in India. There are also rules framed under the provisions of these laws. The following are the laws that are currently in operation in the country:

1. The Poisons Act, 1919

2. The Drugs and Cosmetics Act, 1940 (this was amended various by Drugs (Amendment) Acts in 1955, 1960, 1962, 1964, 1972, 1982 and 1986)

3. The Drugs and Cosmetics Rules, 1945

4. The Pharmacy Act, 1948

5. The Drugs and Magic Remedies (Objectionable Advertisement) Act, 1954

6. The Medicinal and Toilet Preparations (Excise Duties) Act, 1956

7. The Narcotic Drugs and Psychotropic Substances Act, 1985

8. The Drugs (Prices Control) Order, 1995

General legislations that have a significant bearing on pharma industry in the country.

1.   The Industries (Development and Regulation) Act, 1951

2.   The Trade and Merchandise Mark Act, 1958

3.   The Indian Patents and Design Act, 1970.

From among these legislations the following four play a critical role in the development of the industry:

(a) Schedule 'M' of the Drugs and Cosmetic Act 1940

(b) The Indian Patents and Designs Act, 1970

(c) Patents (Amendment) Act, 1999

(d) The Drugs (Price Control) order (DPCO), 1995

These legislations are briefly described so as to appreciate their likely impact on and response from the manufacturers and others concerned.

(a) *Schedule 'M' of the Drugs and Cosmetics Act (1940)*

The Schedule 'M' classifies the various statutory requirements mandatory for all drugs, pharmaceuticals and medical disposable industry relevant as per current good manufacturing practices (CGMP). Schedule 'M' was last revised in 1986, when the concept of GMP was first introduced. The Central Government is now revising the Schedule 'M' to get it "harmonized with that of the various developed and developing countries and also to the level of the well established international organizations such as the World Health Organisation (WHO)".

WHO guidelines on GMP for pharmaceutical products urge that:

*   All manufacturing processes are clearly defined, systematically reviewed, and shown to be capable of consistently manufacturing pharma products of the required quality that comply with their specifications.

- All necessary facilities are provided including qualified trained personnel, adequate premises and space, suitable equipment and services, correct materials, containers and labels, approved procedures and instructions, suitable storage and transport and adequate personnel, laboratories and equipments for in process controls.

- Instructions and procedures are written in clear and unambiguous language.

- Operators are trained to carry out procedures correctly.

- Records are made (manually and/or by recording instruments) during manufacture to show that all the steps required by the defined procedures and instructions have actually been taken and that the quantity and quality of the product are as expected and any significant deviation fully recorded and investigated.

- Records covering manufacture and distribution are retained in a comprehensive and accessible form.

- A system is available to recall any batch of product from sale or supply; and

- Complaints about marketed products are examined, the causes of quality defect investigated, and appropriate measures taken.

A special sub committee constituted by the Government of India has proposed revamping of the Schedule M, covering specifications such as general requirements in case of buildings and premises, personal sanitation and hygiene, training, production and operation controls, quality control and assurance, stability and validation studies, documentation, complaints and self-inspections; and special requirements for individual formulation categories. Among other things, the amendment calls for the following:

- To maintain a ratio of 1:2 between the constructed area and surrounding premises to prevent environmental pollution.

- To install a validated water system to aid monitoring and control of bio-burden levels.

- To have a good disposal system, in the absence of which to have arrangements to recycle rejects.

- To have proper environmental control, with emphasis on buildings, till the primary packaging is complete.

- To ensure supply of filtered air in all production areas to prevent environmental pollution.

- To have specifically designed areas for production, quality control, storage and ancillary areas.

- To take adequate precautions to segregate the manufacture of highly potent drugs to avoid cross contamination.

- To design adequate operational and process controls to ensure reproducible quality of drugs.

- To ensure total quality control from raw materials procurement till the retail counter.

- To undertake detailed stability studies to establish the quality of drugs in different climatic and storing conditions.

- To evolve clear and realistic documentation procedures.

(b)   *The Indian Patents and Designs Act, 1970*

This Act aims at protecting inventions. The term of patent granted is in respect of an invention claiming the method of process of manufacture of a substance. For a medicine or drug the protection is given for a period of five years from the sealing of the patent or seven years from the date of patent, whichever period is shorter. The Controller of Patents, Designs, and Trade Marks appointed under the Trade and Merchandise Act, 1958 is the Controller of Patents.

(c)   *Patents (Amendment) Act, 1999*

After signing the GATT agreement, India needed to change its patent law from process patent regime to a product patent regime. Developing countries are given time till 2005 to change their patent legislation. Since January 1, 1995, India has begun to accept applications for product patents, which go into a black box. This box is to be opened in 2005 to establish right of priority before granting patent. From January 1, 1995 to October 31, 1999, 2994 product patents have been filed for pharmaceutical products. Meanwhile for each such patent application that has been accepted, exclusive marketing rights (EMR) have to be granted for a period of five years.

The Controller of Patents examines the applications to ascertain whether there is a violation of the relevant provisions of Patent Act. The government can not only fix the price of the product covered under EMR, but also reserve the rights to grant compulsory license or revocation of patent. Provision is made to ensure that EMRs are not granted for substances based on Indian System of Medicines where the products are already in public domain.

(d)   *The Drugs (Prices Control) Order (DPCO), 1995*

The DPCO provides for ceiling prices for medicines, the lists of which are reviewed periodically. Over the years substantial changes have been made in the DPCO in terms of reduction in the number of drugs under price control and simplification of application procedures. The DPCO, 1995 allows for exemption from price control for new bulk drugs which have not been produced elsewhere and which are developed through indigenous R and D.

On the recommendation of the Hathi Committee (1973), the Government of India created a Drug Price Equalisation Account (DPEA) under the DPCO. This equalisation is done on the basis of a weighted price average determined by the government. Any company that sells the product at higher margins on account of cheaper sourcing of inputs is held liable to pay up the overcharged amount to the government.

WTO Product patent regime 2005:

From January 2005 product patent regime will come into existence replacing existing process patent regime because of that the companies cannot manufacture products, which have registered patent for a period of seven years. This makes Pharmaceutical manufacturers to invest money in R&D and develop their own drugs and patent them. SMEs who don't have R&D facilities will face problems and end up as jobbers to the big market players.

List of approved associations/societies

1. INDIAN MEDICAL ASSOCIATION
2. INDIAN DENTAL ASSOCIATION
3. BRITISH MEDICAL ASSOCIATION
4. ROYAL SOCIETY OF MEDICINE, ENGLAND
5. ALL INDIA OPTHALMOLOGICAL SOCIETY
6. INDIAN SCIENCE CONGRESS
7. INDIAN PSYCHIATRIC SOCIETY
8. INDIAN ASSOCIATION OF PATHOLOGISTS AND MICROBIOLOGISTS (IAPM)
9. NATIOAL SOCIETY OF MALARIA AND OTHER COMMUNICABLE MOSQUITO BORNE DISEASES
10. TRAINED NURSES ASSOCIATION OF INDIA (TNAT) AND STUDENT NURSES ASSOCIATION OF INDIA (SANI)
11. INDIAN RADIOLOGICAL ASSOCIATION
12. ASSOCIATION OF SURGEONS OF INDIA
13. ASSOCIATION OF PLASTIC SURGEONS OF INDIA
14. UROLOGICAL SOCIETY OF INDIA
15. ASSOCIATION OF THORACIC AND CARDIO VASCULAR SURGEONS OF INDIA
16. BRITISH INSTITUTE OF RADIOLOGY, INCORPORATED WITH ROHTCEN SOCIETY

17. ROYAL SOCIETY OF TROPICAL MEDICINE
18. SOCIETY OF BIOLOGICAL CHEMISTS
19. BOMBAY MEDICAL CONGRESS
20. NEUROLOGICAL SOCIETY O INDIA
21. ASSOCIATION OF PHYSICIANS OF INDIA
22. INDIAN ASSOCIATION OF DERMATOLOGISTS, VENEREOLOGISTS AND LAPROLOGISTS
23. THE SOCIETY OF GENERAL MICRO BIOLOGY OF ENGLAND
24. THE FAMILY PLANNING ASSOCIATION OF INDIA
25. THE BRITISH DENTAL ASSOCIATION
26. THE PHYSIOLOGICAL SOCIETY OF INDIA
27. THE ROYAL MEDCIAL PHYSICOLOGICAL SOCIETY OF INDIA
28. THE INDIAN LEPROSY ASSOCIATION
29. THE INDIAN ASSOCIATION OF HISTORY OF MEDICINE
30. THE INDIAN PUBLIC HEALTH ASSOCIATION OF INDIA
31. THE TUBERCULOSIS ASSOCIATION OF INDIA
32. THE INDIAN MEDCIAL LICENTIATES ASSOCIATION
33. THE INDIAN PHARMACEUTICAL ASSOCIATION
34. ASSOCIATION OF TOLARYNGOLOGISTS
35. INDIAN SOCIETY OF ANAESTHETISTS
36. THE INDIAN PHYSCO THERAPEUTICAL SOCIETY
37. ASSOCIATION OF PHYSCIOLOGISTS AND PHARMACOLOGISTS OF INDIA
38. THE INDIAN ACADEMY OF PEADIATRICS
39. CARDIOLOGICAL SOCIETY OF INDIA
40. THE INTERNATIONAL SOCIETY OF AMERCIAL COLLEGE OF CHEST PHYSICIANS
41. THE INDIAN COUNCIL OF MENTAL HYGINE
42. THE INDIAN ASSOCIATION FOR THE ADNACEMNT OF MEDICAL EDUCATION
43. THE NATIONAL ACADEMY OF MEDICAL SCIENCES

44. THE BRITISH ASSOCIATION OF UROLOGICAL SURGEONS (HOME AND OVERSEAS)

45. THE INDIAN ASSOCIATION FOR CHEST DISEASES

46. THE DERMATOLOGICAL SOCIETY OF INDIA

47. THE ANATOMICAL SOCIETY OF INDIA

48. THE AMERCIAN PSYCHIATRIC ASSOCIATION

49. THE INDIAN CANCER SOCIETY

50. THE COLLEGE OF PATHOLOGISTS (LONDON)

51. THE FEDERATION OF OBESTERIC AND GYNAECOLOGY SOCIETIES OF INDIA AND ITS AFFILIATED LOCAL OBESTERIC AND GYNAECOLOGICAL SOCIETY

52. INTERNATIONAL ASSOCIATION OF ORAL SURGEONS 53. DIABETES ASSOCIATION OF INDIA

53. INTERNATIONAL SOCIETY OF ELECTRIC SLEEP AND ELECTRO ANAESTHESIA

54. INTERNATIONAL FEDERATION FOR MEDCIAL AND BIOLOGISCAL ENGINEERS, LONDON

55. INDIAN HOSPITAL ASSOCIATION

56. INDIAN SOCIETY OF AEROSPACE MEDICINE

57. THE BIOLOGICAL ENGINEERING SOCIETY

58. THE INDIAN SOCIETY OF HEMATOLOGY AND BLOOD TRANSFUSION

59. THE SOCIETY FOR THE STUDY OF INDUSTRIAL MEDICINE, INDIA

60. THE INDIAN SOCIETY FOR THE REHABILITATION OF HANDICAPPED

61. INTERNATIONAL COLLEGE OF DENTISTS

62. INDIAN ASSOCIATION OF CLINICAL PHYCHOLOGISTS

63. SOCIETY OF NUCLEAR MEDICINE OF INDIA

64. INDIAN SOCIETY OF GASTROENTEROLOGY

65. THE INDIAN SPEECH AND HEARING ASSOCIATION

66. THE INDIAN COLLEGE OF ALLERGY AND APPLIED IMMUNOLOGY

67. NUTRITION SOCIETY OF INDIA

68. THE INDIAN ACADEMY OF FORENSIC MEDICINE

69. INDIAN PHARMACOLOGICAL SOCIETY OF INDIA

70. THE MARINE MEDICAL SOCIETY OF INDIA

71. INDIAN SOCIETY OF BLOOD TRANSFUSIONAND IMMUNOHEA-MATOLOGY

72. THE INDIAN ASSOCIATION OF SPORTS MEDCINE

73. THE ENDOCRINE SOCIETY OF INDIA

74. THE INDIAN HOSPITAL PHARMACISTS ASSOCIATION

75. THE INDIAN ASSOCIATION FOR RADIATION PROTECTION

76. THE INDIAN PHYSOLOGICAL ASSOCIATION

77. THE INDIAN PHYSOLOGICAL ASSOCITION

78. THE INDIN ORTHODONTIC SOCIETY

79. THE AMERCIAN PHYSIOLOGICAL SOCIETY

80. THE ASSOCIATION OF CLINICAL BIOCHEMISTS OF INDIA

81. THE ASIAN SOCIETY OF COLORECTAL SURGERY

82. THE INTERNATIONAL COLLEGE OF SURGEONS (INDIAN SECTION)

83. INDIAN ACADEMY OF CYTOLOGISTS

84. ASSOCIATION OF MEDICAL PHYSICISTS OF INDIA

85. ASSOCIATION OF ORAL AND MAAXILO-FACIAL SURGEONS OF INDIA

86. ALL GOVERNMENT LABORATORIES UNDER CSIR

87. INDIAN SOCIETY OF PERIODONTOLOGY

88. INDIAN ASSOCIATION OF MEDICAL MICROBIOLOGISTS (IAMM)

89. INDIAN ASSOCIATION OF PHYSICAL MEDICINE AND REHABILITATION

90. INDIAN COUNCIL OF MEDCIAL RESERACH (ICMR)

91. ANY MEDCIAL COLLEGE/UNIVERSITY IN INDIA

92. MEDCIAL COUNCIL OF INDIA (MCI)

93. WORLD HEALTH ORGANISATION

94. BURNS ASSOCIATION OF INDIA

95. NATIONAL ASSOCIATION OF CRITICAL CARE MEDICINE (INDIA)

96. THE INDIAN ASSOCIATION OF GYNAECOLOGICAL ENDOSCOPSITS

97. INDIAN SOCIETY OF SURGICAL ONCOLOGY (ISO)

98. THE BIO MEDCIAL ENGINEERING SOCIETY OF INDIA
99. INDIAN SOCIETY OF HEALTH ADMINSTRATORS
100. THE ORTHOTICS AND PROSTHETICS SOCIETY OF INDIA
101. INDIAN ASSOCIATION OF MEDICAL STATISTICS (IASM)
102. INDIAN ASSOCIATION FOR TH ESTUDY OF SEXUALLY TRANSMITTED DISEASES
103. INDIAN ASSOCIATION OF PREVENTIVE AND SOCIAL MEDCINE
104. ASSOCIATION OF INDUSTRIAL PSYCHIATRY OF INDIA
105. ACADEMY OF HOSPITAL ADMINISTRATION
106. GERIATRIC SOCIETY OF INDIA
107. COMPTER SOCIETY OF INDIA
108. RESERACH SOCIETY OF ANAESTHESIOLOGY AND CLINICAL PHARMACOLOGY
109. INDIAN ORTHOPEADIC ASSOCIATION
110. INDIAN VIROLOGICAL SOCIETY
111. INDIAN SOCIETY OF NEPHROLOGY
112. INDIAN SOCIETY FOR SURGERY OF THE HAND
113. INDIAN RHEUMATISM ASSOCIATION
114. INDIAN CHEST SOCIETY
115. INDIAN SOCIETY OF ORGAN TRANSPLANTATION
116. ASSOCIATION OF MEDCIAL BIO CHEMISTS OF INDIA
117. NATIONAL NEONATOLOGY FORUM
118. HOSPITAL INFECTION SOCIETY – INDIA
119. INDIAN SOCIETY OF HOSPITAL WASTE MANAGEMENT
120. INDIAN EPILEPSY SOCIETY
121. INDIAN ACADEMY OF ECHO CARDIOGRAPHY
122. INTERNATIONAL TRAUMA ANAESTHESIA AND CRITICAL CARE SOCIETY (INDIAN SECTION)
123. INDIAN SOCIETY OF VASCULAR AND INTERVENTIONAL RADIOLOGY
124. INDIAN SOCIETY OF OTOLOGY

SUMMARY:

Governance in pharmaceutical industry means to understand the associations, societies and statutory councils which monitor and control the functioning and performance of the pharmaceutical companies. The Pharmacy education and profession in India up to graduate level is regulated by the PCI, a statutory body governed by the provisions of the Pharmacy Act, 1948 passed by the Parliament. The dynamic growth of Indian Pharma Industry, a knowledge based industry, and the recommendations of four major Pharmaceutical associations made the Ministry of Commerce & Industry to realize the need for separate export promotion council. Accordingly, Pharmaceuticals Export Promotion Council (PHARMEXCIL) has been set up. Organisation of Pharmaceutical Producers of India (OPPI) established in 1965, is a premier association of research based international and large pharmaceutical companies in India and is also a scientific and professional body. Details about some pahrama associations like Bulk Drug Manufacturers Association (India), Indian Drug Manufacturers' Association (IDMA) are dealt.

Finally medical detailing is an educational activity by sales representatives– 'detailers'–e.g., from pharmaceutical companies or manufacturers of medical devices, to provide details or scientific information on a product's potential uses, benefits. e-detailing is the use of the internet as the medium of communication for pharmaceutical sales detailing of physicians. It is a pharmaceutical or medical device firm-sponsored, internet-based program that informs prescribers about products or diseases using digital technology. Therefore many formats are possible including use of technologies. such as the internet, video-conferencing and interactive voice conferencing for enabling the interaction with the physician

REVIEW QUESTONS

1. Explain the objectives and functional procedures of Pharmacy council of India?

2. What is the constitution and composition of Pharmacy council of India/

3. Discuss any three pharmaceutical associations and their role in promoting pharmaceutical industry in India?

4. What are the roles and responsibilities of a pharmaceutical professional?

5. Discuss the principles and ethics to follow by a pharmaceutical professional?

6. What is medical detailing? Explain the objectives of it.

7. What is e-detailing process? What are the various types of e-detailing and their features?

8. Explain various legislations that govern the manufacture and sale of drugs and pharmaceuticals in India.

Chapter 8

DRUG STORE MANAGEMENT

8.1 INTRODUCTION

Drugstore and pharmacy are the same terms commonly being used, but drug stores are not always required to have a pharmacist if they only sell medicine but not make them.

In pharmacies they can prepare prescription medicine. The drugstore is the place where you can buy aspirin, shampoo, toilet paper and a coke; they also have a pharmacy where you buy the prescription drugs.

8.2 DRUG STORE

A temporary location for drug and disposable surgical items needed for operational purposes, and should be planned, organized and operated in such a way that the period of residence of each item is as short as possible consistent with economic operation.

RESPONSIBILITIES

- Economy (Space Vs Cost)
- Identification (Stores code)
- Receipt (Accepting stores)
- Inspection (Quality & Quantity)
- Issue and Dispatch (Receiving demand & handing over to users)
- Stock records (Bin cards & Ledgers)

PRINCIPLES OF DRUG STORE ADMINISTRATION

I. The "Five Plus Five Rights" of Drug Administration
   ive Traditional Rights

      A. Right client

      B. Right drug

      C. Right dose

      D. Right time

      E. Right route

Five Additional Rights

A. right assessment

B. right documentation

C. client's right to education

D. right evaluation

E. right to refuse

A.   Right Client

Nurse must do:

- ❖   verify client → check ID bracelet & room number
- ❖   have client state his name
- ❖   distinguish bw 2 client's with same last names

B.   Right Drug

- ❖   medication order may be prescribed by:
  - a.   Physician
  - b.   Dentist
  - c.   Podiatrist
  - d.   Advanced practice registered nurse (APRN)
- ❖   Components of a drug order:
  1.   date & time the order is written
  2.   drug name (generic preferred)
  3.   drug dosage
  4.   frequency & duration of administration
  5.   any special instructions for withholding or adjusting dosage
  6.   physician or other health care provider's signature or name if TO or VO
  7.   signature of licensed practitioner taking TO or VO

- ❖   **Nurse must do:**
  - •   check med order is complete & legible.
  - •   know general purpose or action, dosage & route of drug
  - •   compare drug card with drug label **three times**.

1. at time of contact with drug bottle/ container
2. before pouring drug
3. after pouring drug

❖ Categories of Drug Orders:

1. Standing Order / Routine Order
   - ongoing order
   - may have special instructions to base administration
   - include PRN orders ex. digoxin 0.2 mg PO q.d., maintain blood level at 0.5 – 2.0 ng/ml

2. One-time (single) order
   - given only once, at a specific time ex. Cefixime 2mg IM at 7 AM on 12-1-05

3. PRN order
   - given at client's request & nurse's judgement for need & safety ex Mefenamic Acid 500mg q 4h PRN for pain

4. STAT order
   - given once, immediately ex. Morphine 2mg IV STAT

C.   Right Dose

❖ **Nurse must do:**
- Calculate and check drug dose accurately.
- Check PDR, drug package insert or drug handbook for recommended range of specific drugs.
- Check **heparin, insulin and IV digitalis** doses with another nurse.

❖ Stock- method vs Unit-dose method

D.   Right Time

❖ **Nurse must do:**
- Administer drugs at specified times.
- Administer drugs that are affected by foods, before meals.
- Administer drugs that can irritate stomach, with food.
- Drug administration may be adjusted to fit schedule of client's lifestyle, & activities. & diagnostic procedures.

- Check expiration date.
- Antibiotics shld be administered at even intervals.

E.   Right Route

❖ **Nurse must do**:
- assess ability to swallow before giving oral meds.
- Do not crush or mix meds in other substances before consultation with physician or pharmacist
- Use aseptic technique when administering drugs.
- Administer drug at appropriate sites.
- Stay with client until oral drugs have been swallowed.

F.   Right Assessment

❖ get baseline data before drug administration.

G.   Right Documentation

❖ Immediately record appropriate info
- Name, dose, route,time & date, nurse's initial or signature

❖ Client's response:
- narcotics
- analgesics
- antiemetics
- sedatives
- unexpected reactions to meds.

❖ Use correct abbreviations & symbols.

H.   Right to Education

❖ Client teaching :
- therapeutic purpose
- side-effects
- diet restrictions or requirements
- skill of administration
- laboratory monitoring

❖ Principle of Informed Consent

I.   Right Evaluation

- ❖ client's response to meds.
  - o   effectiveness
  - o   extent of side-effects or any adverse reactions.

J.   Right to Refuse

- ❖ **Nurse must do:**
  - • determine, when possible, reason for refusal.
  - •   facilitate px's compliance.
  - • explain risk for refusing meds & reinforce the reason for medication.
  - • Refusal shld be documented immediately.
  - • Head nurse or health care provider shld be informed when omission pose threat to px.

Medication Misadventures include:

1. administration of wrong medication & IV fluid.
2. incorrect dose or rate
3. administration to the wrong patient
4. incorrect route
5. incorrect schedule interval
6. administration of known allergic drug or IV fluid
7. omission of dose or discontinuation of med or IV fluid that was not discontinued.

II.   Guidelines for Correct Administration of Medications

A. Preparation

1. Wash hands before preparing meds.
2. Check for allergies.
3. Check medication order with physician's orders, medicine sheet, & medication card.
4. Check label on drug container 3 times.
5. Check expiration date on drug label.
6. Recheck drug calculation with another nurse.
7. Verify doses of drugs that are potentially toxic with another nurse or pharmacist.

8. With unit dose, open packet at bedside after verifying client identification.

9. Pour liquid at eye level.

10. Dilute drugs that irritate gastric mucosa or give with meals.

B. Administration

11. Administer only those drugs that you have prepared.

12. Identify the client by ID band or ID photo.

13. Offer ice chips when giving bad tasting medicine.

14. Assist client to appropriate position.

15. Provide only liquids allowed on the diet.

16. Stay with client until meds are taken.

17. Administer no more than **2.5 to 3 ml** of solution by IM at one site.

18. Infants receive no more than **1 ml** of solution by IM at 1 site & no more than **1 ml** subcutaneously. NEVER recap needles.

19. Give drugs last to client who need extra assistance.

20. Discard needles & syringes in appropriate containers.

21. Follow appropriate drug disposal based on institution policy.

22. Discard unused solutions from ampules.

23. Store appropriately unused solutions from open vials.

24. Write date & time opened & initials on label.

25. Keep narcotics in a double-locked drawer or closet. Med cart – locked at all times when nurse is not around.

26. Keys to narcotics drawer must be kept by the nurse & not stored in drawer.

27. Avoid contamination of one's own skin or inhalation to minimize chances of allergy.

C. Recording

28. Report drug error immediately to nurse manager & physician. Complete an incident report.

29. Charting: record drug given, dose, time, route & your initials.

30. Record drugs promptly after given, esp STAT doses.

31. Record effectiveness & results of meds given, esp PRN meds.

32. Report to physician & record drugs that were refused with reason for refusal.

33. Record amount of fluid taken with medications on input & ouput chart.

Behaviors to Avoid During Medication Administration:

- Do not be distracted when preparing meds.
- Do not give drugs poured by others.
- Do not pour drugs from containers whose labels are partially removed or have fallen off.
- Do not transfer drugs from one container to another.
- Do not pour drugs into the hand.
- Do not give expired medications.
- Do not guess about drugs & drug doses. Ask when in doubt.
- Do not use drugs that have sediment, are discolored, or are cloudy (& shld not be).
- Do not leave medications by the bedside or with visitors.
- Do not leave prepared medications out of sight.
- Do not give drugs if the px says he has allergies to the drug or drug group.
- Do not call the px's name as the sole means of identification.
- Do not give drug if the client states the drug is different from drug he has been receiving. Check the order.
- Do not recap needles. Use universal precautions.
- Do not mix with large amount of food or beverage that are contraindicated.

III.   Forms & Routes for Drug Administration

A. Tablets & Capsules

- oral meds not given to patients who are:
  - o   vomiting
  - o   lack gag reflex
  - o   comatose
- Do not mix with large amt of food or beverage or contraindicated food or infant formula
- **Enteric- coated & timed-release capsules must be swallowed whole.**
- Administer irritating drugs with food to lessen GI discomfort.
- Administer drugs on empty stomach if food interferes with absorption.
- **Drugs given sublingually must remain in place until fully absorbed.**
- Encourage use of child-resistant caps.

B. Liquids

- Forms : elixir, emulsions, suspensions
- read label if dilution or shaking is required.
- **read the MENISCUS.**
- refrigerate once reconstituted.

C. Transdermal

- systemic effect
- more consistent blood levels & avoid GI absorption problems associated with oral products.
- **patches should NOT be cut.**

D. Topical

- Applied to skin with a glove, tongue blade or cotton - tipped applicator.
- Apply to clean dry skin when possible.
- Do not contaminate the medication in a container.
- Do not "double dipped" .
- Observed sterile technique when skin is broken.
- Use firm strokes if medication is to be rubbed in.

E. Instillations

- Eyedrops
    1. wash hands
    2. lie or seat down and look up towards ceiling
    3. remove any discharge by wiping out from inner canthus
    4. rest hand holding the dropper against the client's head.
    5. gently draw skin down below affected eye to expose conjunctival sac
    6. administer drops into center of the sac
    7. gently press lacrimal duct with sterile cotton ball or tissue for 1 to 2 mins after instillation
    8. keep eyes closed for 1 to 2 mins following application

- Eye Ointment
    1, 2, 3, 4,- same as above

5 . squeeze strip of ointment (abt ¼ inch, unless stated otherwise).

5. keep eyes close for 2-3 mins.

6. instruct px for blurred vision for a short time.

7. apply at bedtime, if possible.

- Ear Drops

    1. wash hands.

    2. medicine should be at room temp.

    3. sit up with head tilted slightly toward unaffected side.

    4. child: **pull auricle down & back**. (above 3yr ,same as adult)
    adult: **pull up & back.**

    5. instill prescribed drops.

    6. do not contaminate dropper.

    7. maintain position for 2-3 minutes.

- Nose Drops & sprays

    1. have client blow nose.

    2. tilt head back for drops to reach frontal sinus. tilt head to affected side to reach ethmoid sinus.

    3. Administer prescribed number of drops or sprays. Some sprays, close 1 nostril, tilt head to closed side & hold breath or breathe thru nose for 1 minute.

    4. Keep head tilted backward for 5 minutes after instillation.

F. Inhalations

- Semi-fowlers or high-fowler's position.
- Teach correct use of nebulizer & metered-dose inhalers.

STOCK CONTROL IN PHARMACY

The operation of continuously arranging flows of medicines so that stock balances are adequate to support the current rate of consumption, with due regard to economy. The following table gives details of typical hospital pharmacy areas and operations.

Hospital Pharmacy Operations

Pharmacy Area	Key Terms	Questions
Hospital Pharmacy Services		What are ways of classifying hospitals? What are the functions of a hospital? What services provided by a hospital pharmacy are similar to community pharmacy services? What services are unique to the hospital pharmacy?
Inpatient Drug Distribution Systems		How is the drug distribution system in a hospital different from processing medication orders in the community pharmacy?
Unit Dose Packaging	Unit dose	Why do hospitals use unit dose packaging?
Repackaging Medications		When might repackaging medications be necessary? What materials are used for repackaging? What is the purpose of a repackaging control log, and what information does it contain?
Medication Orders	Medication fill list unit dose profile	What is the procedure for processing and delivering medication orders in the hospital pharmacy? How are orders for controlled substances processed and delivered? What information is on a unit dose label?
Floor Stock	Floor stock	What types of medications are typically kept in floor stock? Give examples. What are advantages and disadvantages of the floor stock system for filling medication orders? What are the pharmacy technician's duties and responsibilities in regard to floor stock?
Intravenous Admixture Service	Total parenteral nutrition (TPN)	Why is it better to prepare IV solutions in the central pharmacy rather than on the hospital floor? When is TPN used?
Clinical Services	Satellite pharmacy protocol	In addition to dispensing drugs, what clinical services might a hospital pharmacy provide? Give examples of how a specialty trained clinical pharmacist might function as part of a medical team. What is a pharmacokinetics consult service? Why are pharmacy technicians important to a hospital pharmacy's ability to provide clinical services?

Pharmacy Area	Key Terms	Questions
Drug Information Services	Formulary	What things must be considered in preparing a hospital formulary? How does the inventory of drugs in a hospital pharmacy differ from that of a community pharmacy? What are the duties and responsibilities of the drug information pharmacist? What tasks might a pharmacy technician who works in the hospital's drug information center perform?
Outpatient Pharmacy Services		Whom does a hospital outpatient pharmacy generally serve?
Automation in the Hospital Pharmacy	Stat medications	How is automation used in the hospital pharmacy? What are advantages of using automation?
Inventory Management	Investigational drugs	What procedure is used to purchase hospital pharmaceuticalsWhy is the source of drug products changed infrequently? What might be the pharmacy technician's duties and responsibilities in regard to inventory management? In addition to controlled substances, what other type of pharmaceuticals requires special inventory management?
Organization of the Hospital		How is the administration of a hospital organized? How does the hospital pharmacy fit into this organization?
Pharmacy Administration		What are the duties and responsibilities of the director of pharmacy? What pharmacy services might be outsourced?
Joint Commission on Accreditation of Healthcare Organizations	Joint Commission on Accreditation of Healthcare Organizations (JCAHO) accreditation	Why is JCAHO accreditation so important to a hospital? In addition to hospitals, what facilities does JCAHO evaluate? Describe the JCAHO accreditation process
Safety-Related Standards		What safety issues involve the hospital pharmacy?
Quality of Care Standards		What are JCAHO's National Quality Improvement Goals? How does JCAHO determine how well a hospital meets these goals? How is the hospital pharmacy involved in the National Quality Improvement Goals?

Pharmacy Area	Key Terms	Questions
Pharmacy and Therapeutics Committee	Pharmacy and therapeutics (P&T) committee	What is the chief responsibility of the P&T committee? What is the purpose of a hospital formulary? In addition to listing specific drugs, how else might a formulary restrict the prescribing of drugs in the hospital?
Infection Control Committee	Infection control committee (ICC) nosocomial infection sharps universal precautions	With what type of infection is the ICC primarily concerned? What are ways in which the ICC might carry out its responsibilities? List universal precaution guidelines. With what type of exposure are pharmacy personnel usually the most concerned?
	Institutional review board (IRB) informed consent	What is the chief responsibility of the IRB? What should an informed consent document include? How might the pharmacy and pharmacy technician be involved in an investigational study?

Pharmacy, as practiced in the hospital setting, is developing a wide spectrum of clinical services which have become part of the overall pharmaceutical services although it may not be directly associated with drug dispensing. Fundamental to these clinical services is the pharmacist's knowledge of drugs, diseases, patient and drug variables, and his ability to interact closely on a personal basis with other health professionals and patients. Academic training in areas such as toxicology, pathophysiology and therapeutics, as well as clinical experience, provide the background for a pharmacist to function in this clinical role. The service includes:

1. Drug information, which encompasses the collection, organization, retrieval, interpretation and evaluation of the applicable literature inappropriate fashion

2. Collection of the pharmacy patient data base

3. Patient education

4. Monitoring and auditing of therapeutic regimens

5. Drug-use review

6. Monitoring/reporting of specific adverse drug reactions to decrease their incidence and

7. Performing other similar functions designed to improve patient care by maximizing drug use. Clinical functions may also extend to the pharmacist's role in primary care as well as in the management of chronic care patients.

8.3 ORGANIZATION

The hospital pharmacy should be properly organized meeting the minimum requirements prescribed by the Bureau of Food and Drugs (BFAD), the Licensure Act of the Bureau of Licensing and Regulations (BLR), and the enhancement standards of the HOMS based on the capabilities of hospitals. The organization of a hospital pharmacy must satisfy the needs of the pharmacists performing their role as the vital link in the chain of health providers dedicated to patient care.

The hospital Pharmacy Service shall be under the general supervision of the administrative officer or Chief of Hospital (COH); it will directly be administered and supervised by a licensed pharmacist. The organization serves to establish the authority relationships between positions and to assign special tasks that achieve the pharmacy's objectives. The pharmacy head practices the five essentials of good management, namely, planning, organizing, directing coordinating and controlling.

An organizational chart showing the flow of administrative authority is essential to the selection and categorization of employees. The chart should be designed to meet the specific requirements of the Pharmacy Service. (See Figure). In addition to the chart, an outline showing the subdivisions of the service and the responsibilities assigned to each subdivision may also be prepared for larger pharmaceutical services. (See Figure) It is imperative to list all functions of the Pharmacy Service in the planning of personnel requirements of various work systems (e.g., a unit dose system will require more personnel for dispensing in-patient drugs than a floor stock system); the estimate of work load units per function (e.g., a number of outpatient prescriptions, number of drug information requests, etc.); the time required to complete each workload unit, etc.

Figure: Pharmacy service –position chart

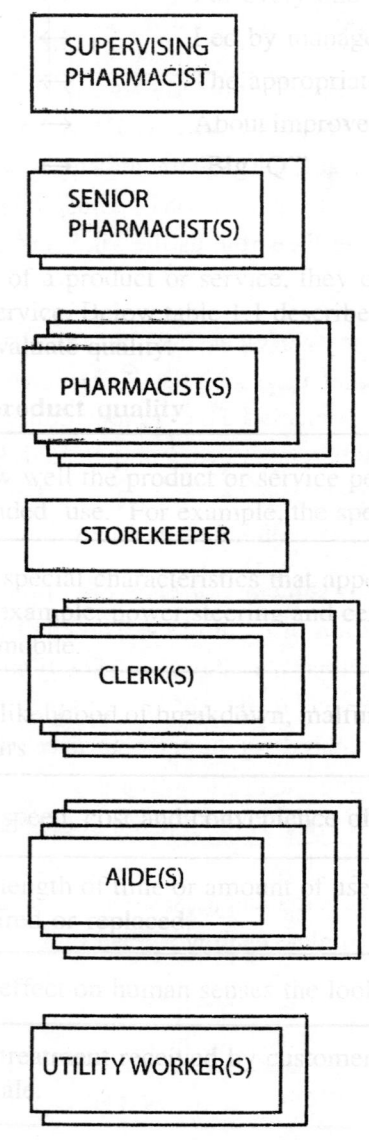

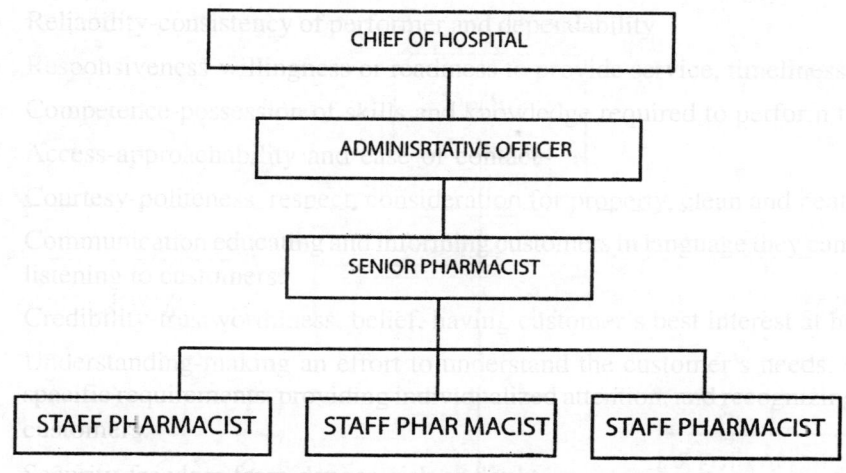

Figure: Secondary level (25 beds)

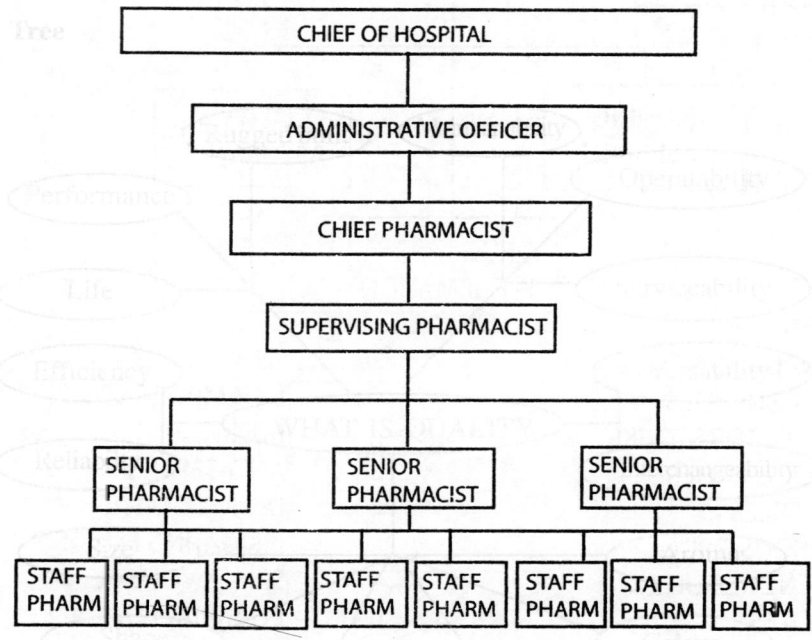

Figure: Tertiary level (200 beds)

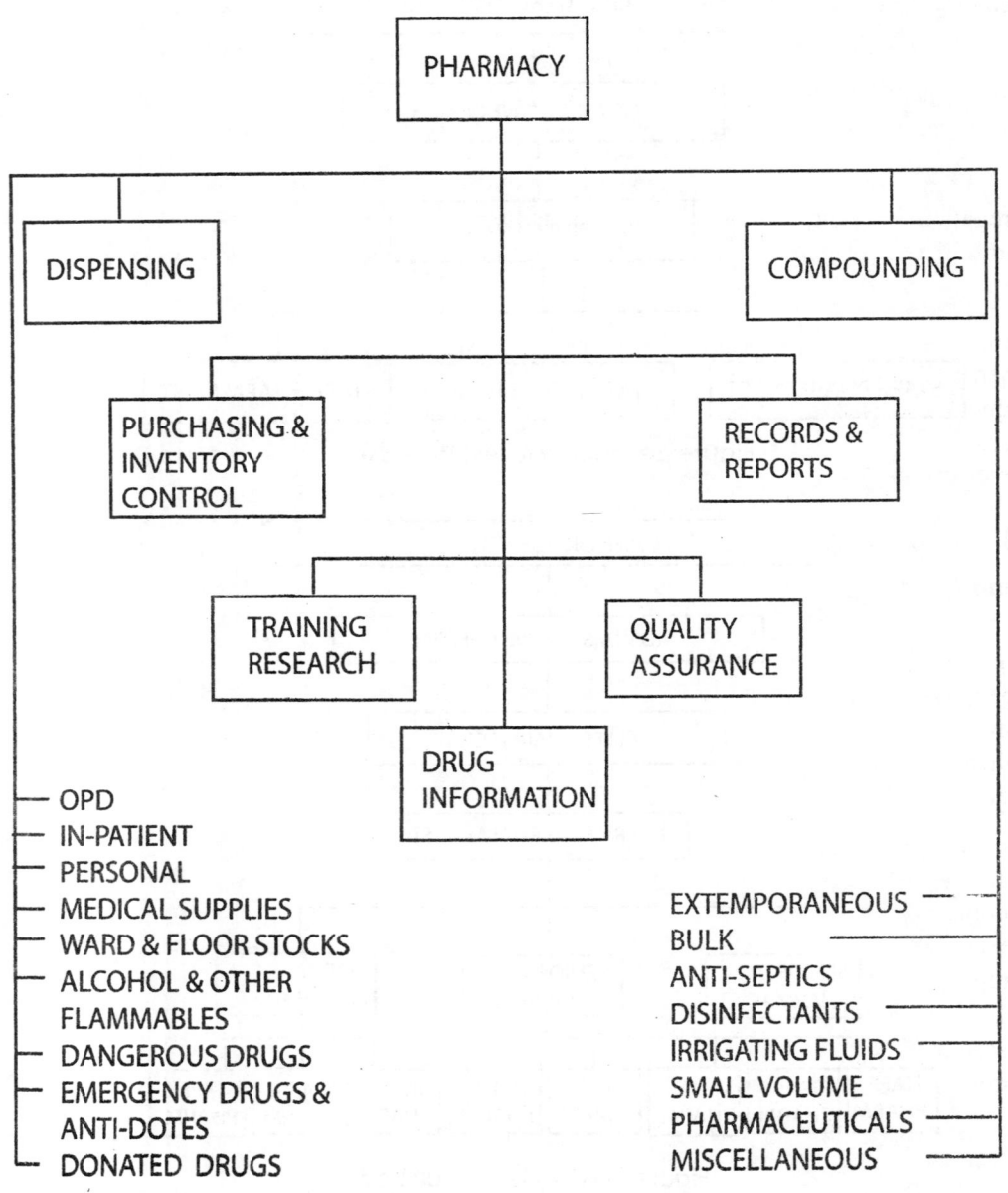

PHARMACY

DISPENSING

COMPOUNDING

PURCHASING & INVENTORY CONTROL

RECORDS & REPORTS

TRAINING RESEARCH

QUALITY ASSURANCE

DRUG INFORMATION

- OPD
- IN-PATIENT
- PERSONAL
- MEDICAL SUPPLIES
- WARD & FLOOR STOCKS
- ALCOHOL & OTHER FLAMMABLES
- DANGEROUS DRUGS
- EMERGENCY DRUGS & ANTI-DOTES
- DONATED DRUGS

EXTEMPORANEOUS
BULK
ANTI-SEPTICS
DISINFECTANTS
IRRIGATING FLUIDS
SMALL VOLUME PHARMACEUTICALS
MISCELLANEOUS

PLANTS, FACILITIES, EQUIPMENT AND OTHER MATERIALS

Plants, facilities, equipment and other materials of the hospital pharmacy will come under the establishment of the hospital pharmacy. However, these are further standardized based on the hospital's capability levels, size, and scope of service.

Adequate spaces, equipment and supplies are provided for the professional and administrative functions of the Pharmacy Service to assure patient safety through the proper storage, preparation (compounding, packaging and labeling) and dispensing of drugs.

Drugs are stored under proper condition of sanitation, temperature, light, ventilation, segregation and security. The pharmacy must develop a design which would be accessible to both in and out-patients, business offices and frontline services.

Premises must be well-ventilated and should have concrete tiles or wooden flooring. There must be suitable areas for compounding, manipulating parenteral medications, dispensing, adequate storage of drugs with wooden pallets for drug boxes and biological products as specified in the label, for flammables and for administrative functions. It must be provided with suitable cabinets for storing poison and/or dangerous drugs with sectional type of cabinets and must have an adequate supply of water.

8.4   COMMUNITY PHARMACY ADMINISTRATION:

Community Pharmacies

The Community Pharmacy denotes the Pharmacy services in the Community centers for general public. The **Community Pharmacy Division** aims to offer healthcare to group of people with emphasis on prescription and related matters including the medication. The Community Pharmacists are the most accessible source of information about drugs, medication and related aspects. The concept of Community Pharmacy is very developed in other countries.

The community pharmacist procures and dispenses prescription drugs, provides advice about OTC drugs, and communicates information between the patient and physician as appropriate. The amount of contact a community pharmacist has with a patient varies greatly. The community pharmacist also screens for drug-drug and drug-disease interactions, therapeutic duplication, and adherence to drug regimens (by examining the pattern of drug refills or directly questioning the patient). Patients should be encouraged to fill all of their prescriptions at the same pharmacy and, when possible, to get to know their pharmacist; this approach enables the pharmacist to oversee their drug therapy comprehensively.

Many community pharmacists are available for face-to-face patient counseling and usually provide take-home printed material. Some community pharmacists participate in disease management programs, with emphasis on preventive medicine. In this role, the pharmacist must complete a certificate program in one or several disease states that are widely prevalent in the elderly (e.g., diabetes mellitus, heart failure, hypertension, incontinence, osteoporosis) and, electively, in areas such as immunization awareness (eg, counseling susceptible patients to obtain vaccination against influenza and pneumococcal pneumonia). In several states, pharmacists can administer influenza vaccines. Community pharmacists may also offer screening and monitoring programs (e.g., for BP or plasma glucose).

The process of community pharmacy system include patient interaction, prescription processing, filling, prescription handling & delivery to patient and secondary patient interaction as shown in the figure

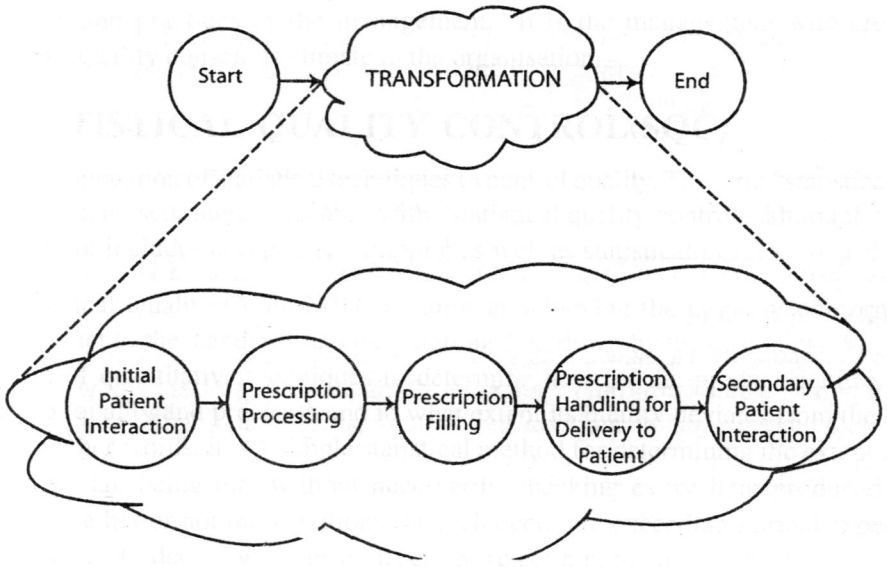

Figure. Operations performed in a community pharmacy to fill prescriptions.

Health is a word very familiar to us but it also carries a lot of complications and problems. According to the World Health Organisation, health is a state of complete physical, mental and social well-being and not merely absence of any illness. To make the above definition of health practical we have to depend upon a "health care team".

A health care team is the group of people who share a common health goal and common objectives determined by community needs. India with the greatest cultural diversity, health though an important issue is being neglected due to many hindrances. The condition is further worsened due to insignificant drug use problems. On the spurge of many spurious, duplicate and adulterated drugs, it is in the hands of the pharmacist particularly the community pharmacist, to take up the challenge for providing better health care and better outcomes economically.

Role of community pharmacist

A community pharmacist is the professional who would be in direct access to the public and whose duties are widely sought after by the public and patients. He dispenses medicines with a prescription and in certain cases without a prescription where applicable (OTC drugs). As he is the person who will be in direct contact with the public, he has to play an important role in decreasing the mortality and morbidity in the public.

Community pharmacy practice evolved in the post second World War period. A pharmacist not only began to perform functions that were new to pharmacy, but they began to innovate functions and make original contribution to literature. The popular motto of "patient oriented practice" and "drug use control" came into practice. But unfortunately the role of community pharmacist is not so much recognized till today especially in India and needs strong efforts.

Although community pharmacist is of key importance in providing better healthcare, it is the matter of shame for us that the Indian patient does not find any difference between the grocer and the pharmacist. Despite of major role of community pharmacy, the situation and condition of the community pharmaceutical service has stood where it was like a man walking on a treadmill. He walks and walks and sweats, but remains in the same place. Until and unless the link between the people and physician i.e. the pharmacist does not get its proper recognition any dreams of making India, a healthier nation cannot be fulfilled.

The need of the hour is to make community pharmacist a key towards better health care. The community pharmacist can take part in health promotion campaigns, locally and nationally, on a wide range of drug related and health related topics. A community pharmacist involvement could play an important role in the following areas of health care.

Nutrition Counseling

Community pharmacist can make, significant contributions in assuring adequate nutrition by advising his patients about basic food needs, keeping to correct improper food habits in children, advising on special requirements, suggesting special diet instructions for diabetic patients and people with food allergy and participating in school lunch programs and schemes like mid-day meals etc. in rural areas.

There are certain facts such as women who often eat fish or omega-3-fatty acids are less likely to suffer stroke, symptoms of hyper vitaminosis result in irregular menstrual cycle and excessive intake during pregnancy may cause birth defects. The pharmacist can tell these facts to people to ensure better health. Now a days designer foods i.e. nutraceuticals/

dietary supplements have not only gained considerable acceptance but also have newfound use and applications. They are considered to provide medical or health benefits. The community pharmacist could explain these new innovative products and their standardization.

Women Welfare-Pregnancy and Infant Care

A famous Sanskrit Shloka from Manusmriti scriptures goes as "Yatra Nariyastu Poojayanta, Ramante Tatra Deva" which means, "where women are worshipped Gods preside there". Women are the corner stone for effective public health and investing in women translate into investing in family, community and the Nation. Against the backdrop of a hectic and demanding schedule, women's health receives the least priority when it should be the first.

A woman goes through different stages throughout her life, each of which has specific need and the presence of a counselor is needed in each one of them. The pharmacist who understands the normal course of pregnancy and infancy is at a distinct advantage as he or she can guide the mother in simple matters of hygiene and management. The community pharmacist can encourage breastfeeding and can play a major role by guiding the mother for the protection of the child by following proper immunization schedule. Efforts are definitely underway in this area. The US FDA's office of women's health has created "women's health: take time to care", a national public awareness campaign, where apart from giving information about safe medicine use, they also hold local interactive sessions led by pharmacists and other health care professionals.

Rational Use of Drugs

A community pharmacist can also advise on the administration of the medication, provide information on the storage of the medication and wherever necessary he can counsel the patient. Education regarding the disadvantage of polypharmacy can also be given to the patient. Drug information system should be set up and access to adverse drug reaction system should be made. A community pharmacist should do therapeutic drug monitoring and he should have a sound knowledge of genotype reporting i.e. predictive pharmacology.

Drug information awareness programmes should be conducted to make people aware of side effects of certain OTC drugs e.g. Aspirin - a wonder drug also has many side effects like gastric ulceration; asthma and large doses may cause tinnitus. Regular use of paracetamol can cause harm to the liver. How many amongst the common people know that drugs such as Action 500, Coldarin can increase blood pressure in patients having hypertension. Even pain shows difference between men and women. Where women respond better to the opiods such as morphine, pentazocine and pethidine men respond better to the non-steroidal anti-inflammatory drug, ibuprofen. Considering the above examples, in the best interest of public health a community pharmacist can provide counseling to common people unaware of these side effects.

Moreover the definition of an OTC product should be that "which does not require the prescription of a registered medical practitioner but which can be sold only under the supervision of a pharmacist". In a nut shell there should be rational use of drug i.e. right drug in right patient in right dose at right time. A community pharmacist is one of the inevitable members of the health care team who can help to achieve the goal of rational use of drugs by following good pharmacy practices. It is found that interventions by pharmacists in explaining the patients about medicines prescribed to them can significantly enhance patient knowledge of correct use of medicines from 56 per cent to 90% per cent.

There is yet another role of the community pharmacist in India and that is enhancing the availability of essential drugs. Nearly 70% population in India is deprived of essential drugs for a variety of reasons including non-availability of health professionals and improper professional advice about the usage of drugs.

In India, one pharmacist for two thousand persons can improve access to medicines and their safe utilizations. The existing pool of community pharmacist can become an important instrument in bringing about this change. For setting higher standard for pharmacy practice in the country the essential drug list should be received by the government and the availability of the essential drugs should be enhanced through the pharmacists.

Sexually Transmitted Diseases-AIDS

India has 3.5 million HIV positive cases, which is about 10% of the global HIV cases and barely second to South Africa. HIV drugs are expensive and beyond the reach of common man. Huge resource of community pharmacist can educate people in the prevention and information of HIV/AIDS. For this, Federation of Indian Pharmacists project in India on involvement of pharmacist in fight against AIDS is very relevant.

Another sensitive issue is the increasing number of women patients suffering from AIDS. The number rose from 7% in 1985 to 18% in 1995. Although many classes of antiretroviral are available like protease inhibitors, nucleoside reverse transcriptase inhibitors and non-nucleoside reverse transcriptase inhibitors, patients need close monitoring and strict dietary regimen. Explaining to what HIV is, its transmission, risk reduction, patient counseling are the components of the counseling that a community pharmacist can provide.

Alcohols, Drug Abuse and Smoking Cessation

The diseases of alcoholism and drug abuse also come under the preview of the community pharmacist. The pharmacist has a key role to help individuals who become dependent upon alcohol. Drug abuse is similar to alcoholism yet different because it has been gaining more acceptances among young people. Annual mortality from tobacco use exceeds that from all other causes combined. Smoking is the greatest single preventable cause of morbidity and mortality in India. It is the responsibility of a community pharmacist to take an active role in helping the smokers to stop smoking. Following a number of smoking policies through out the pharmacy, by written information and posters, can do this. The pharmacist can advise on the products available to assist the patient in giving up smoking. Counselling sessions can be made by the community pharmacist to stop smoking.

Family Planning

One of the greatest needs of the hour is to control the tremendously increasing population in India. A community pharmacist is the one who can control this rising population by counseling with people and doing programmes which exhibit the problems related with large families. He can tell the various families planning measures that are available in the market at affordable prices. He can educate the people and convince them about the advantages of having small families. So, like all other aspects community pharmacist plays a very important role in this case also.

Individualization of Drug Therapy

Today the latest concept in medicine is towards individualization of drug therapy. Where judicious patient care is needed individualization of drug therapy becomes a need, and a pharmacist can play a vital role in this. A physician who is preoccupied with patient diagnosis and treatment may not spare time for patient counseling regarding pharmaco-economics, drug information, alternative therapy, moral supporting etc. A pharmacist can set up a separate consultation room and provide counseling to the patient. He can store the details of patient history, allergies and other details necessary for therapy so that the concept of individualization of drug therapy could be implemented.

The ideal frontline pharmacist of the future has been described as a seven star pharmacist-some one who is equal in excellence to a five star hotel yet accessible to everyone from the richest to the poor. The future 7 star pharmacists will have seven principal roles to play:

— Care giver;

— Decision-maker;

— Communicator;

— Leader;

— Manager;

— Life long learner and

— Role model.

The community pharmacist with the above skills and attitudes should make himself an indispensable partner in health care system of a nation.

8.5 DRUG STORE PLANNING:

The two most important considerations for location are heavy customer traffic and minimum competition. As with most other retail establishments, convenience has become the key word. That is, the more a store is a one-stop shopping center for its customers and provides services that save time, the better its chances for survival. Some drug stores have increased their sales by locating in a strip mall near convenience stores, hardware stores, restaurants, liquor-stores, dry cleaning facilities. It has become increasingly difficult for a drug store to remain profitable in a stand-alone site unless it is near a great deal of health care related business, such as a hospital, a nursing home, or a health care complex.

The location of the pharmacy can affect several aspects of operations. The location of the pharmacy can affect the following:

- How easily and efficiently the inputs for operations can be acquired
- How easily the outputs of operations can be transferred to the consumers of those outputs
- Which outputs are chosen to be offered by a given business (designing of goods and services)

In a pharmacy, there are certain skilled positions that need to be taken into consideration when locating the business. Operating a pharmacy in a location that is conducive to attracting qualified pharmacists to work there is important. The pharmacy must also be able to receive deliveries of the various products sold by the pharmacy. Proximity to consumers and the preferences of consumers will play a role in how easily the pharmacy's goods and services are transferred to the consumers of those services. For example, a chain pharmacy in a busy metroplex whose customers rely on public transportation to get to the pharmacy to have their prescriptions filled will be greatly inconvenienced if the pharmacy does not have in stock all the medications necessary to fill their prescriptions. This, therefore, affects the operations of the pharmacy. It may cause the pharmacy to have a larger inventory than otherwise needed or a delivery service to minimize the inefficiency or customer dissatisfaction that may result from not being able to fill the prescriptions while patients wait. Or the pharmacy could be located in an area with a large population of people who want to pick up their medications at a drive-through window (e.g., mothers with sick infants). The market factors that are influenced by location will influence the operations of the pharmacy. The goods and services themselves also may make one location more profitable than another.

The design of goods and services is part of operations, and if a business is located near people who want and need its products and services, it may enhance the business's chance of attracting them to the store. For example, a pharmacy located in an ethnic neighborhood that has a population of people who rely on natural products to maintain health might decide to offer such products to those consumers. The proximity of these people to the store and their desire to have such products may increase the chance of those items being profitable for the pharmacy. The location of the pharmacy certainly can affect operations, and so can the location of various goods and services within the pharmacy.

Drug store layout

A pharmacy needs to be designed to maximize the efficiency of the processes conducted to create the goods and services. For example, when filling a prescription, the path that the prescription takes from the patient to the pharmacist who will fill it needs to be efficient. A layout that decreases efficiency is likely to contribute to decreased profitability. Steps that require the prescription to "backtrack in the process" need to be eliminated or minimized by designing an efficient layout. The layout can also affect the efficiency with which services are provided. Having a counseling area that is readily accessible to the pharmacist and patients will increase the efficiency of providing information to patients. And it even may increase the likelihood that patients will ask for information when they need it. In addition to the efficient operations of the pharmacy, the layout of the pharmacy will affect the patients' movement through the store. This has implications for product placement and pharmacy design.

Supply-chain management

The *supply chain* is the chain of businesses that supply pharmacies with necessary inputs. It is important to build relationships and have agreements with other companies that will maximize the efficiency of receiving the goods needed to fill prescriptions. Wholesalers are the primary vendors for pharmacies. They distribute the majority of prescription drugs. Some chain pharmacies receive goods from distributors that they own and also have relationships with wholesalers. This is done so that they can get goods that may not be available from their own distributors or so that they can get goods quickly if the wholesaler delivers more frequently than their own distributors. These relationships need to be established with reputable companies that can provide reliable service particularly in times of need, such as during natural disasters. These relationships can take different forms and entail different levels of service.

By signing a contract with a pharmacy, a wholesaler agrees to provide the pharmacy with products and services that may help the pharmacy to operate efficiently. These services can include electronic order submission, next-day delivery service, private-label programs, cooperative advertising programs, special-handling services, pharmacy computer systems, pricing, and store planning. Management of the supply chain is of great importance in the creation of goods or the provision of services that involve goods. The key elements of the decision in choosing suppliers for the pharmacy are the timely delivery of needed and properly stored medications by a licensed and reputable wholesaler at the best price. In making this decision, there are a number of wholesalers from which to choose.

Some chain pharmacies have regional or local distribution centers that receive medications from the wholesaler in large quantities and repackage the medications into package sizes that are more feasible at the store level.

Large, full-service wholesalers are only one type of wholesaler available to supply pharmacies and other health care institutions with medications. There are also regional wholesalers, smaller wholesalers, and secondary wholesalers.

Good Medical Stores Management

The following are objectives of good medical stores management

- To guarantee a **continuous supply** of drugs and medical supplies.
- To **maintain the quality** of drugs during the whole distribution process.
- To **minimize losses** through expiration and deterioration.
- To **control** theft and corruption.
- To keep accurate inventory **records.**
- To provide stock movement **information** in order to forecast needs.
- To use **transport** means efficiently.

Planning Issues for Hospital Pharmacies with Growing Outpatient Populations

In recent years, there has been an increasing emphasis in healthcare on the provision of ambulatory care services. It is predicted that in the next few years, 80 percent of all healthcare services (including surgery) will be delivered in an outpatient setting. This shift away from acute hospital care is due to several factors. The incentives by managed care have led to a decrease in hospitalization rates and length of stays. Advances in technology have made less invasive procedures possible on an outpatient basis. As ambulatory care services grow, hospitals will be reserved for the most acutely ill inpatients.

As outpatient procedures continue to grow and as hospitals increasingly become the repository for the most acutely ill inpatients, the hospital pharmacy will be in a constant state of transition. These trends will affect the work process in the hospital pharmacy and the storage and handling of pharmaceutical supplies.

Pharmacy space planners will need to become more involved in and understand the issues that impact the relative proportions of storage, work process, and drug distribution spaces in the layout of the pharmacy. Asking the right questions and getting the appropriate answers will contribute to planning a pharmacy layout that will respond to this changing environment.

Areas of Hospital Pharmacy Stores

There are three areas of a "typical" hospital pharmacy which consists of Bulk Stores, Outpatient Pharmacy, and Inpatient Pharmacy.

Bulk Stores

As the number and variety of medications expand to treat more acutely ill patients and to fill the increasing volume and diversity of prescriptions for outpatients, many hospital pharmacies are implementing a just-in-time (JIT) inventory delivery system from vendors. A JIT system supplies items as close to the time of use as possible in an effort to reduce large inventories, decrease space requirements, and lessen financial outlay.

The growth and emphasis on JIT delivery and stock in the pharmacy means there is less volume of individual items, but more deliveries more often. This may reduce the amount of space required for bulk storage, but increase the amount of space needed for vendor bins, carts, pallets, and totes. The clinical work area in Bulk Stores is typically divided into four functions to support inventory management:

- Ordering
- Receiving
- Storing
- Distribution

Ordering

This area provides the link to pharmaceutical vendors for JIT delivery and stock. This requires a number of computers and printers that are linked to these prime vendors and to other areas of the pharmacy for inventory control. Since inventories are kept to a minimum with JIT, they must be monitored closely to ensure adequate supplies are kept on hand. Electrical and data access must be provided for the equipment.

Receiving

In the "breakout area," supplies are removed from their outer containers or vendor bins. This process will require a large work table, preferably mobile and height-adjustable. Space should be allotted for receptacles used for packaging materials sorted for recycling.

In addition to this work center there should be a hand-washing sink, a storage area for JIT vendors, and a large reusable trash receptacle on casters. If bar codes are not supplied by vendors, they may be applied to the stock here. This may require a separate workstation for a computer and the bar coding equipment as well as storage for bar coding supplies.

Storing

General Storage: After the items are "broken" out of their outer containers, they are stored in the general storage area. Pharmaceuticals must be separated and stored by category (for example, orals, topicals, liquids, eye drops, ear drops, vaginals, nasal sprays, injectables, etc.). Expiration dates of perishable drugs must be considered, and stock rotated as required. A separate area also is required to hold outdated, obsolete, or recalled pharmaceuticals that need to be returned to vendors. This requires shelving of various depths and heights to accommodate the variety of items that need to be separated by category. General storage will also require a refrigerator, a freezer, and utility carts for moving supplies throughout the pharmacy.

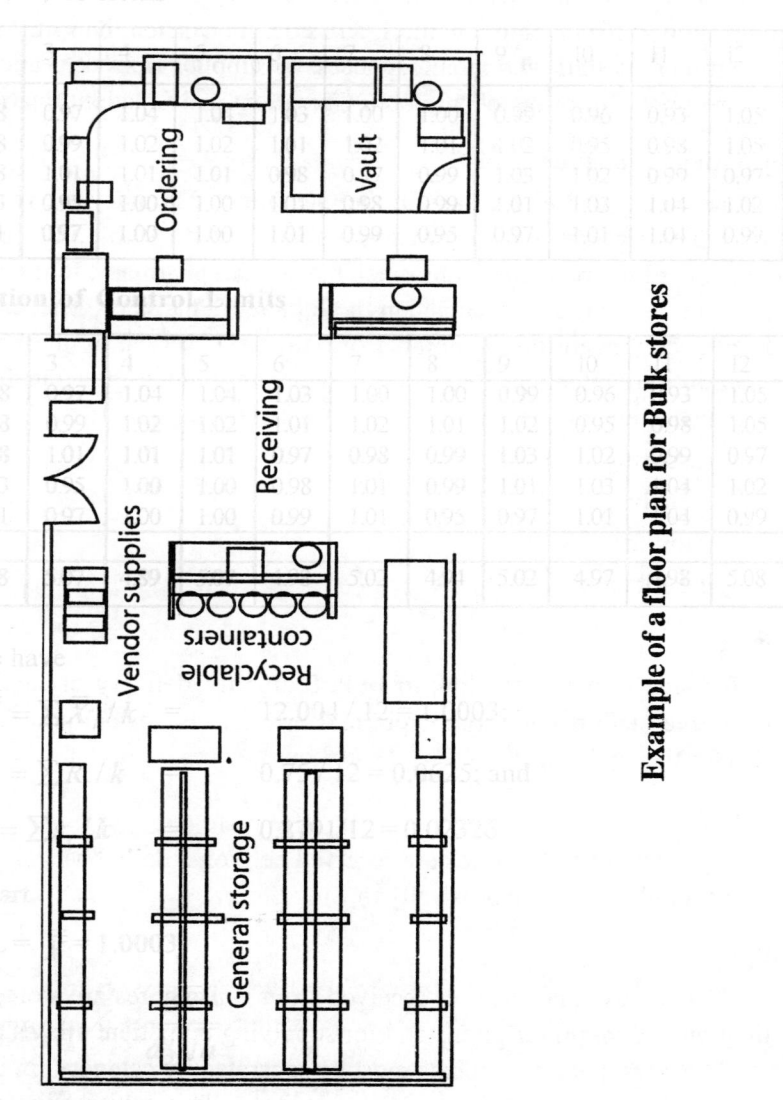

Example of a floor plan for Bulk stores

Controlled Substance Storage: Narcotics and other government-controlled substances are stored in a vault or locked room in the pharmacy, usually located away from the primary entrance, but in a highly visible location. The vault is a separate room with walls and a door to restrict access to controlled substances with schedules II through V. Schedule II narcotics remain inside the vault until needed. Daily supplies of schedule III through V narcotics may be removed from the vault and stored in a secure area in both the Outpatient and Inpatient Pharmacies. Within the vault there may be a refrigerator, a workstation with computer support for inventory control, and storage. Outside the vault, a small workstation may accommodate staff who monitors access to supplies from the vault. Distribution Bulk Stores is responsible for restocking both Outpatient and Inpatient Pharmacies.

2. Outpatient Pharmacy

Pharmacists and technicians in the Outpatient Pharmacy are responsible for filling outpatient prescriptions and for providing pharmacy stock to clinics and off-site centers. The Outpatient Pharmacy functions much like a retail pharmacy. It has completely different products and distribution systems than the Inpatient Pharmacy. The size of the Outpatient Pharmacy is contingent on the number of outpatients served by the hospital. The clinical work area in the Outpatient Pharmacy is typically divided into four functions to support inventory management:

- Ordering
- Receiving
- Storing
- Distribution

Ordering

This area provides the link to Bulk Stores for delivery of stock. This requires an administrative station with computers and printers. Electrical and data access must be provided for the equipment.

Receiving

Supplies from Bulk Stores are received here on a daily basis or several times a day. This area should be in close proximity to Bulk Stores.

Storing

Active Stores: The supplies received from Bulk Stores are stored here and are used for filling outpatient prescriptions and for supplying outpatient clinics and off-site centers. As in Bulk Stores, pharmaceuticals must be separated by category (orals, topicals, liquids, eye drops, ear drops, vaginals, nasal sprays, etc.). This will require shelving of various depths and heights to accommodate the variety of items that need to be separated by category. This area will also require a great deal of space to store the volumes of paper products needed to fill prescriptions – printer paper, prescription labels, prescription bags, warning labels for containers, as well as hard copies of prescriptions.

Manufacturing: The manufacturing area provides, when requested, the compounding and manufacturing of special prescriptions for outpatients that are not available commercially. This area requires a work counter, computer, storage cabinet, and sink with an area for drying glassware

Prepackaging: In the prepackaging area, medications in both liquid and tablet form are divided and packaged as needed in smaller containers for outpatient use. Manufacturing and Prepackaging may be located in a self contained room.

Distribution

Order Entry: Prescriptions come into order entry as hard copies at the dispensing windows (handed from patient to pharmacy staff), electronically via computers (from physician to pharmacy staff), or by automated phone-in system (from patients requiring refills). This information is input into the computer system where it is checked for warnings of interactions with other drugs and for potential allergic reactions by the patient. Once these warnings are cleared, the computer generates a label on a printer with the name of the patient and medication required. The size of this area and the number and layout of stations will be impacted by how the prescription information is received. Work space will require computers, printers, telephones, fax machines and/or scanners, and some paper storage. Some pharmacies utilize a computerized queuing system to triage the prescription information – triggering the sequence of filling prescriptions based on priority factors. This requires an administrative support station for computers and printers.

Filling: Fill lines are workstations where pharmacists or technicians manually fill prescriptions. At the beginning of the fill line, the prescription label is used as the "picking list." The container is filled with the appropriate items, and at the end of the fill line the pharmacist checks the filled prescription against the computer and does a visual check as well. The filled prescription is put into a paper bag which is placed alphabetically on shelving close to the dispensing window. Each fill line may have two computers, one linked to order entry to print the prescription labels, the other, used by the pharmacist, to check the accuracy of the filled prescriptions. Fill lines require a work counter with shelving for storage of fast moving items along with shelves and bottle drawers below the work surface. The number of fill lines and computers will be determined by the number of outpatient prescriptions needed to be filled.

The fill station can assume different configurations. If the work performed at the fill area needs to be separated from patient contact, the configuration is often a straight line located away from the order entry/dispensing window. This results in more privacy for the staff and may speed up the time necessary to fill prescriptions. If the pharmacy wishes to promote patient contact between staff and patient, the configuration may take the form of a pod. This is often an L-shaped workstation. One staff member enters the order, fills the prescription from shelving located next to the window, and dispenses it to the patient.

This configuration offers the most privacy for the patient and promotes consultation. Fill lines accomplish 80 percent of the filling, but there are other work counters that need to be accommodated. Controlled substances require a separate work counter with locked storage. This area is typically located away from the fill line to facilitate the privacy and concentration required. The preparation of suspensions requires a sink and distilled water. Here the staff adds a predetermined amount of water to a powder to create a suspension. Some pharmacies may also require chemotherapy stock. This station will require a hazardous waste receptacle.

The growth of outpatient services means larger stocks of medications. As a result, many pharmacies use automated counting/dispensing systems to fill prescriptions faster and more accurately. Some of these systems are floor mounted, while others may need work surface support. These systems require shelving to hold separate stock with special manufacturers' numbers that the equipment can recognize. Innovations in technology also have enabled the use of robotics to replace the staff time spent on tedious and repetitive functions, as well as increase the accuracy of filling. This speeds up the medication delivery time and frees the pharmacist to spend more time with patients. Robotics equipment takes up additional floor space, which may be limited in some existing facilities. There also needs to be space allotted for storage of repair parts for maintaining the equipment and separate stock with special manufacturers' numbers that the robotics can recognize. Robotics have unique requirements for utilities – gas, air pressure, and electrical.

Dispensing: Dispensing windows are for outpatient prescription drop-off and pick-up. The number of windows required depends on the volume of outpatient prescriptions that need to be processed.

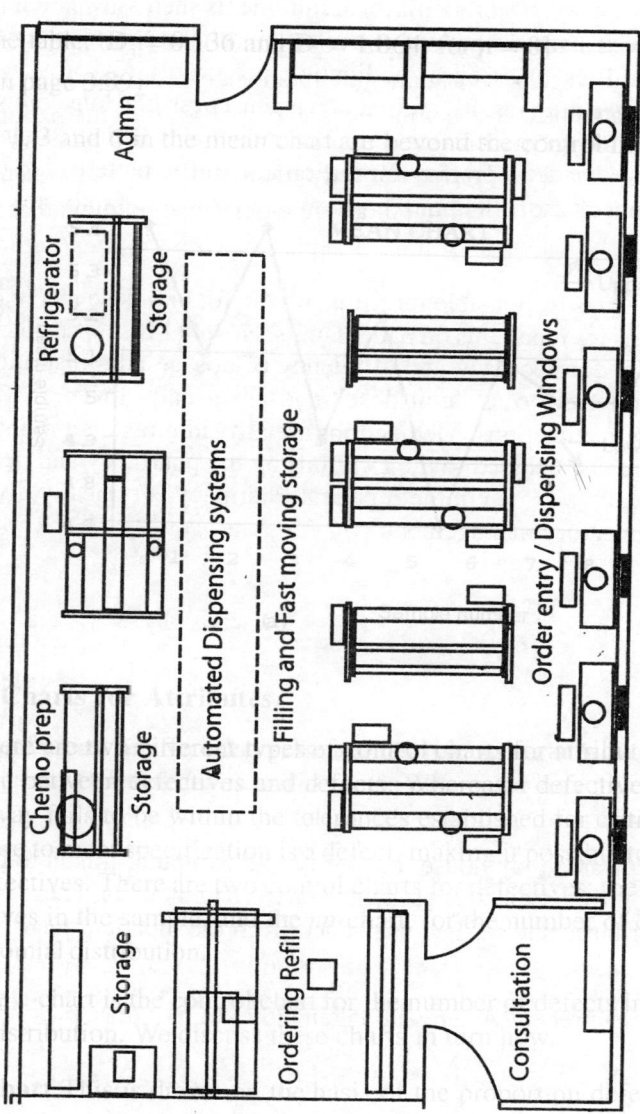

Example of a floor plan for Out Patient Pharmacy

As a general rule, eight windows will support a maximum volume of 12,000 to 14,000 prescriptions per month. The windows should be positioned to support patient confidentiality and address ADA (Americans with Disabilities Act) requirements such as wheelchair access. Administrative space is needed for outpatient consultation where pharmacists can meet with patients and their families to discuss medication programs, give instructions in administration, explain expected drug results, and caution against possible drug complications. A separate, enclosed consultation room increases patient confidentiality in discussing illnesses, drug treatments, and financial matters. Traffic congestion and traffic patterns are becoming more complex as patient consultations within the pharmacy grow at a rapid rate.

3. Inpatient Pharmacy

The Inpatient Pharmacy is responsible for filling orders for unit dose medications and intravenous (IV) medications for inpatients on patient units. Hospital-dispensed medications are packaged in single doses for accuracy and efficiency of dosage administration. These single-dose packages are referred to as "unit dose" and are usually the most frequently ordered or high-volume-use medications. Medications are also administered in intravenous (IV) fluids. These medications are added to the IV fluids by the pharmacy and delivered to the patient units. The clinical work area in the Inpatient Pharmacy is typically divided into four functions to support inventory management:

- Ordering
- Receiving
- Storing
- Distribution

Ordering

Active Stores: This area provides the link to Bulk Stores for delivery and stock. This requires an administrative station with computers and printers. Electrical and data access must be provided for the equipment.

Patient Unit Support: This area may house the mainframe computer linked to automated dispensing machines for controlled substances located on the patient units. These inventories are monitored on a regular basis and refilled as needed from the inpatient pharmacy.

Receiving

Supplies from Bulk Stores are received here and taken either to unit dose picking or to IV/admixture storage.

Storing

Supplies for unit dose picking are stored in the picking stations. IVs are stored in the IV/admixture rooms.

Manufacturing: The manufacturing area provides, when requested, the compounding and manufacturing of special prescriptions for inpatients that are not available commercially.

This area requires a work counter, computer, storage cabinet, and sink with an area for drying glassware.

Prepackaging: In the prepackaging area, bulk medications are divided and packaged as unit dose for inpatient use. Manufacturing and Prepackaging may be located in a self contained room.

Distribution

Order Entry: Order entry is the "communications hub" of the pharmacy and is often in a central or front location. In this area, written medication orders are received and reviewed by the pharmacists. Orders are compared with the patient's medication history or profile to prevent the administration of antagonistic or duplicated drugs. All hard copies of orders are generally stored in this area. Work space must be provided for several staff, as well a sufficient file and equipment space (telephones, computers, printers, paper shredder, fa machine, and copy machine).

Unit Dose Picking: The need for the retrieval of the most frequently used medications in an efficient, time-saving manner has led to the development of the unit dose picking station. This workstation provides a space of limited dimensions containing a maximum quantity of drugs and allows the pharmacist or technician to "pick" the appropriate drugs. Orders can be filled with little wasted time and motion by having high-volume or fast-moving drugs within an arm's length.

The unit dose picking stations can be planned in many different configurations based on space parameters, number of drugs to be dispensed, additional functions and equipment within the station, and the number of staff using the station. Picking stations require storage space for pharmaceuticals separated by category (orals, ingestibles, and topicals). They also need work surfaces where the unit dose can be filled and checked. Typically, there are carts for organizing and containing the stock for delivery to patient units and small mobile work surfaces that can be positioned where needed.

IV Admixture: A specific area of the pharmacy is designated for the function of adding medications to IV fluids prior to administration to the patient. The process of preparing IVs may also be known as sterile preparation of parenteral products or IV admixture. The IV/admixture area requires a large refrigerator, freezer, and generally two carts – one to hold a supply of IV bags and one for delivery to the hospital. The injection of medications into IV fluids is carried out under a horizontal or vertical airflow hood. A large work counter is needed near the hoods for checking the IVs. Also required is a sink with an eyewash station and storage area for IV additives. IV/admixture may also have its own order entry station with computers, printers, and fax machine. Although code requirements may differ, the IV/admixture area must be the cleanest part of the department. It is usually in a closed room with positive pressure for isolation and cleanliness in preventing contamination.

Some facilities are required to utilize a Class 10,000 clean room for IV preparation that is free of contaminants and in which micron-sized particles are screened out. This type of clean room can effectively remove viable microbes by removing particles (less than or equal to 0.5 microns) from standing surfaces and incoming air. This air purity is achieved through the creation of a shell or secluded area that is sealed off from the rest of the environment. As the census of hospitals becomes populated with increasingly more ill inpatients, IV/admixture use will increase. IVs will be infused with more complicated, expensive, and perishable drugs such as biotech drugs, hyper alimentation, and the mix of several drugs in one IV.

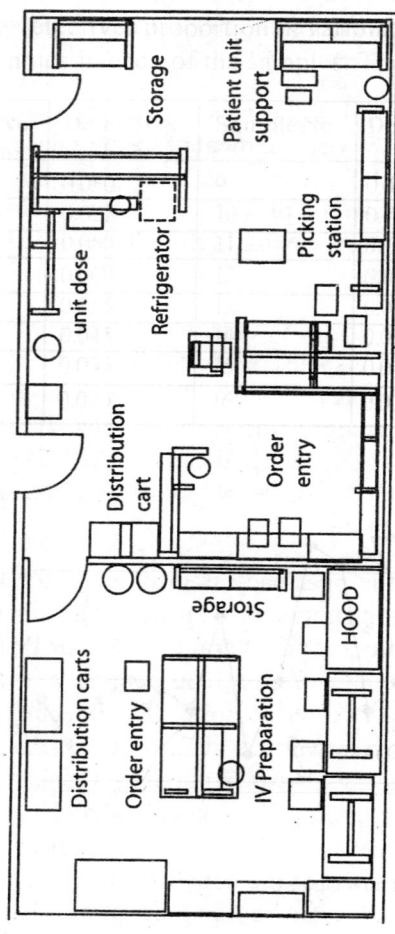

Example of a Floor plan for a Inpatinet Pharmacy

8.6 SALESMANSHIP

Salesmanship is one of the promotional activities of marketing. It is an art of winning the confidence of the customers. It is a technique of convincing a person to buy the goods. Salesmanship is the ability to induce people to buy goods, which they require. It is the ability to convert human needs into wants. The salesman is to help the consumer. In other words, salesmanship is an art of influencing or persuading people to buy the goods.

I. Definition of Salesmanship

According to W.G. Carter, "Salesmanship is an attempt to induce people to buy goods". According to Prof. Stephenson "Salesmanship refers to conscious efforts on the part of the seller to induce a prospective buyer to purchase something that he had not really decided to buy, even if he had thought of it favourably. It consists of persuading people to buy what you have for sale and in helping them to make up their minds." According to the National Association of Marketing Teachers of America, 'It is the ability to persuade people to buy goods or services at a profit to the seller and benefit to the buyer.'

II. Difference between salesmanship and personal selling

Personal selling and salesmanship are often used interchangeably. Personal selling is a broader concept .Salesmanship may or may not be an important part of personal selling.

III. Importance of Salesmanship

In the present day, salesmanship plays an important role. A salesman is the connecting link between sellers and buyers at every stage, i.e., from the collection of raw materials to the finished product. The expansion of the market, growing competition etc., invites a better salesmanship.

a. To Producers

Salesmanship is essential for producers for pushing products into the competitive market. To capture new market also, salesmanship is very important, Salesman increases the sales volume. It brings larger profits to the manufacturers. A salesman works as the "eye and ear" for the manufacturers. They improve their products according to the taste of the consumers and also their sales policies by keeping in mind the suggestions, impression and complaints of the consumers. Salesmanship increases the rate of turnover and hence reduces stock. It minimises the economic stagnation. Consumers can select the best products according to their requirements, taste and preferences.

b. To Consumers

A salesman educates and guides the consumers. He gives them more satisfaction. A salesman helps the consumers in making the right decision and proper selection of the products, which they want to buy.

Promotion may be defined as "the co-ordination of all seller initiated efforts to set up channels of information and persuasion to facilitate the scale of a good or service." Promotion is most often intended to be a supporting component in a marketing mix. Promotion decision must be integrated and co-ordinated with the rest of the marketing mix, particularly product/ brand decisions, so that it may effectively support an entire marketing mix strategy. The promotion mix consists of four basic elements. They are:-

1. Advertising

2. Personal Selling

3. Sales Promotion, and

4. Publicity

   1. Advertising is the dissemination of information by non-personal means through paid media where the source is the sponsoring organization.

   2. Personal selling is the dissemination of information by non-personal methods, like face-to-face, contacts between audience and employees of the sponsoring organization. The source of information is the sponsoring organization.

   3. Sales promotion is the dissemination of information through a wide variety of activities other than personal selling, advertising and publicity which stimulate consumer purchasing and dealer effectiveness.

   4. Publicity is the disseminating of information by personal or non-personal means and is not directly paid by the organization and the organization is not the source.

SALESMANSHIP PROCESS

Salesmanship is the process of applying three way management process (planning, implementation and evaluation) to sales force and its activities. Sales executive begin by setting sales goals and planning sales force activities. This involves forecasting sales, preparing sales budgets, establishing sales budgets establishing sales territories and setting sales quotas.Then the sales force must be organized, staffed, and operated to implement the strategic plans and reach the goals that were set. The final stage involves evaluating the performance of individual's sales people as well as appraising the total sales performance.

EFFECTIVE SALESMANSHIP

Effective salesmanship starts with a qualified sales manager. Finding the right people for the right job is not easy. In many organizations the common practice when the sales management position becomes available is to reward the most productive sales person with a promotion. The assumption is that, as a manager, an effective sales person will be able to impart the necessary wisdom to make. However, the qualities that lead to effective salesmanship are often the opposite of the attributes of successful salesperson. Probably

the other equally successful sales person. Probably the biggest difference in the position is that sales people tends to be self motivated and self reliant, they often work independently, receiving all the credit or blame for their successes or failures. In contrast, sales manager must work through and depend on others, and must be prepared to give recognition rather receive.

To be effective the sales manager must understand customers, appreciate the role of the sales people, and have the respect of the sales force. These attributes can only be required by spending time in sales. Advertising is salesmanship. Its principles are the principles of salesmanship. Successes and failures in both lines are due to like causes. Thus every advertising question should be answered by the salesman's standards. The only purpose of advertising is to make sales. It is profitable or unprofitable according to its actual sales.

It is not for general effect. It is not to keep your name before the people. It is not primarily to aid your other salesmen. Treat it as a salesman. Force it to justify itself. Compare it with other salesmen. Figure its cost and result. Accept no excuses which good salesmen do not make. Then you will not go far wrong.

SALESMANSHIP AND ADVERTISING

The difference is only in degree. Advertising may appeal to thousands while the salesman talks to one. It involves a corresponding cost. Some people spend $10 per word on an average advertisement. Therefore every ad should be a super-salesman. A salesman's mistake may cost little. An advertiser's mistake may cost a thousand times that much. Be more cautious, more exacting, therefore. A mediocre salesman may affect a small part of your trade. Mediocre advertising affects all of your trade. Many think of advertising as ad-writing. One must be able to express himself briefly, clearly and convincingly, just as a salesman must. But fine writing is a distinct disadvantage. So is unique literary style. They take attention from the subject. They reveal the hook.

Successful salesmen are rarely good speech makers. They have few oratorical graces. They are plain and sincere men who know their customers and know their lines. So it is in ad writing. Many of the ablest men in advertising are graduate salesmen. The best we know have been house-to-house canvassers. They may know little of grammar, nothing of rhetoric, but they know how to use words that convince.

8.7 SALES PROMOTION

Sales promotion is one of the most loosely used terms in the marketing vocabulary. We define sales promotion as demand. Stimulating devices designed to supplement advertising and facilitate personal selling. In other words, sales promotion signifies all those activities that supplement, co-ordinate and make the efforts of personal selling and advertising more effective. It is non recurrent in nature which means it can't be used continuously.

Concept of Sales Promotion

Sales promotion consists of diverse collection of incentive tools, mostly short-term designed to stimulate quicker and / or greater purchase of a particular product by consumers or the trade. Where as advertising offers a reason to buy, sales promotion offers an incentive to buy. Sales promotion includes tools for consumer promotion (for example samples, coupons, prizes, cash refund, warranties, demonstrations, contest); trade promotion (for example buying allowances, free goods, merchandise allowances, co-operative advertising, advertising and display allowances, dealer sales contests); and sales-force promotion (for example bonuses, contests, sales rallies).

Sales promotion efforts are directed at final consumers and designed to motivate, persuade and remind them of the goods and receives that are offered. Sales persons adopt several techniques for sales promotion. Creative sales promotion can be very effective. It is the marketing manager's responsibility to specify promotion objectives and policies.

Definitions of Sales Promotion

According to American Marketing Association " Those marketing activities other than personal selling advertising and publicity that stimulate consumer purchasing and dealer effectiveness such as display shows and exhibitions,demonstrations and various non-recurrent selling efforts not in the ordinary routine."

W.J. Stanton defines sales promotion as all those activities other than advertising, personal selling, public relations and publicity that are intended to stimulate customer demand and improve the marketing performance of sellers.

8.8 ACCOUNTING RECORDS IN DRUG STORES

Accounting records in drug stores will normally consists of cash/bank, receipts/payments, journal vouchers, etc. Various books of accounts, such as cashbook, bankbook and ledgers, can be generated and maintained using this module. It can also generate trial balance, balance sheet, and profit and loss statements.

Indent books:

For the purpose of accounting of stores two separate indent books will be maintained in each ward/department, one each for demand of stores on medical stores and dispensary respectively. Quantity of items to be demanded will be fixed every year by the concerned officers based on the average monthly consumption during the preceding twelve months.

Indents will be prepared in TRIPLICATE. All THREE copies will be sent to the Medical Stores. After endorsing the quantity issued on all the three copies of the indent, TWO copies will be sent back to the concerned ward / dept after retaining the original copy in the Medical Store. One of the copies sent to the ward/dept will be sent back to the Medical Store as the 'RECEIPTED COPY' after the actual quantity issued is thoroughly checked by the Nursing in charge and found correct in all respects. The Medical Store will keep all such receipted copies attached with the original copies of the indents for accounting and maintenance of expense ledgers.

Medical stores/dispensaries will issue the stores showing quantities issued on all three copies of the indent against each item. Wards/departments will arrange collection from medical stores/dispensary. Items not issued will be clearly marked as 'NA' and quantity issued column will not be left blank under any circumstances.

Urgent Indents: Indenting of drugs / expendables through urgent indents will be restricted only to the ICU/CCU and other Acute Wards. All other wards / departments must plan their normal indents meticulously so that the need of urgent indents is completely eliminated.

Indenting of Drugs for Super-speciality Centers/wards (Oncology/Renal Transplantation/Endocrinology etc): Indents for drugs like Anti-cancer drugs and drugs used in super-specialized centers will be sent to the Medical Stores ONE day in advance so that the drug is made available to the patient in the morning of the day of initiation / continuation of next phase of therapy.

Indenting of selected / expensive drugs: Certain selected expensive drugs will be indented along with a Case Summary of the patient(s) signed by the Medical Officer . The Case Summary should contain the following details:-

(a)   Particulars of the patient

(b)   Diagnosis

(c)   Very brief justification of the drug to be used for that particular patient.

(d)   Dosage schedule of the indented drug in detail.

Such Case Summaries are intended to ensure justified and realistic indenting of expensive drugs, prevent hoarding and subsequent pilferage of such drugs.

Drugs nearing expiry: All wards / departments will intimate the stock position of all drugs / expendables to the Medical Store which are about to expire, at least three months before their printed date of expiry, which are unlikely to be consumed within this period, so that necessary disposal can be arranged and loss to the state is avoided.

Inventories of non-expendable stores issued to all wards and departments will be maintained in duplicate, one copy with the ward/department and other with the medical stores. Both copies will be signed by the Officer-in-charge ward/department and Medical Stores in charge.

Broadly the following are the accounting records maintained in drug stores:

1. Maintain All Ledger and Cash Book Registers

2. Ledger of all Transaction of Credit And Debit of particular account generate Automatically. Under any account head daily transaction can be generated.

3. Billing and payments are directly associated to account any time balance sheet, Ledger of different heads- party ledger & trial balance can generate

4. Security can be applied to any ledger or balance sheet at any level

5. Balance Sheet (Daily/Monthly/Yearly)

6. Daily receipt/ Payment report / Department wise collection

7. Journals /Cash Book/Bank Book/Sale Book/Purchase Book

8. Registers and Credit Note/Debit Note, / Financial Budget

Financial accounting

The Financial Accounting deals with Cash/Bank, Receipt/Payments, Journal Voucher and General Ledger etc. Books like Cashbook, Bankbook and Ledger book can be generated. This generates reports like Trail Balance, Balance Sheet and Profit and Loss statement.

The Financial Accounting describe about the Account Payable, Account Receivable and General Ledger. Also describe the activities related to IP, OP, bank related activities and provision to clearing the supplier Invoice and keep track of the Account Receivable and Revenue related activities. The services that are covered by the sponsor companies, Insurance Agencies, Family Accounts, Individual Accounts, sponsorship details of the patient, Health Card Insurance are recorded in the system.

- General Ledger, Account Payable and Account Receivable
- Chart of accounts
- Journal Voucher entries
- Customer invoicing
- Cheque (Bank) /cash receipt from customers Invoice receipts matching
- Supplier invoicing
- Cheque (Bank) /cash payments to suppliers
- Advance payments to suppliers
- Credit notes and Debit notes
- Balance sheet, profit and loss account and trail balance
- Asset definition and categorization
- Asset depreciation, transfer, revaluation and write off

- Profit & Loss And Trading Account
- Transaction Vouchers
- Journal : Listing Of Vouchers
- Bill wise Sales / Purchase Vouchers
- Cash Book
- Multicolumn Cash/Bank Book
- Bank Book
- Bank Interest Calculation
- Day Account Balances
- Current Balances
- Account Receivable and Payables
- Ledger
- Trial balance
- Analysis of Accounts
- Month wise Business Indicator
- Month wise Account Balances
- Periodic Account Movements
- Transactions in Accounts
- Account Heads Comparison
- Cash Flow - Movement of Cash
- Fund Flow - Assets Vs. Liability
- Month wise Profit & Loss And Trading Account

Accounts Receivable / Payable

This maintains on-line information of trade creditors and debtor's outstanding. The module maintains bill-wise outstanding information and provides age-wise outstanding reports in detail and summary forms for efficient control on outstanding of the hospital.

Payroll

This module maintains a database of employees in the hospital. The module provides user definable formula setting for various earnings and other standard deductions. The Income tax module captures the sections of income tax and employees investment details.

General Stores

This module maintains on-line information of receipts & issues of items at general stores. The module allows setting up of multiple stores. The module captures the consumption of various cost centers in the hospital.

Purchase Management

The module captures purchase orders raised by the hospital with various vendors. The module provides the tracking of a purchase order till the material is received and cost is accounted in the system. The re-order level, safety quantity and economic order quantities ensure that there is no under-stocking of critical items. The history on supplier's performance and vendor information provides useful MIS.

Patient Billing

Documents that are maintained for patient billion include, health insurance sponsor details Health plans, covered services, applicable rates and discounts, Health plans and covered diagnostic codes, Health plan co-payment details, Sponsor invoicing, Patient billing and collection, Financial postings to Financial account

Payroll

Payroll will include Employee personal details, Leave and attendance management, Loans and advances management, Employee promotion, transfer and resignation and Payroll processing

Pharmacy Store

This deals with all medical items. This module helps in maintaining Item Master Maintenance, Receipt of Drugs/consumables, issue handling of material return, generating retail bills, stock maintenance. It also helps in fulfilling the requirements of both IPD and OPD Pharmacy.

8.9 OPTIONS FOR RETAIL PHARMACIES

Pharmacy chains can choose between ready-to-deploy products, custom built products or buying out source code and customizing it for their requirements. The right choice will depend on factors like size, geographical spread and complexities of each organization. Their current state with respect to system sophistication and process standardization are also important considerations. Some critical factors that must be considered from the economic and implementation perspectives include:

1. Effort and cost involved in developing/purchasing the base version
2. Effort required to deploy the base version across a number of stores

3. Development of user training modules and ease of transition

4. Estimated long term maintenance effort and costs

5. Effort and documentation for support team to stay abreast of developments

6. Flexibility and ease of enhancements for future business needs

7. Ability to run different versions in production, test and development for different' environments and different applications

Pharmacy chains competing for growth in the face of significant competitive challenges face a dire need to improve productivity (to cope with the severe shortage of trained pharmacy staff) and revenue (in the light of reducing reimbursements from insurance and government). To address these challenges, the need is for streamlined operations aligned with their business objectives. As proven by leading Pharmacy chains, selecting the right Rx workflow system can provide a definitive competitive edge in the marketplace.

Pharmacy Management Systems

1. To enable operational efficiency across the chain, managements need to deploy the right-fit pharmacy management system. With adequate due diligence and the right implementation approach, these systems can help with

2. Addressing the shortage of pharmacists by streamlining and automating the workflow process steps. The system should aim for efficient filling of prescriptions while freeing up pharmacists for customer consultation and allowing technicians time for value- added activities

3. Streamlining operations through data sharing across store locations allowing patients to order / refill their Rx from any store. Significant improvement is possible in this area with workload balancing and remote / distributed operations.

4. Segmentation of work process for efficient division of labor

5. Systemic data checks to scan impact of drug combinations or drug allergies to ensure patient wellness and provide counseling to improve relationships with the patient Enhancing customer satisfaction levels and repeat business through timely and consistent customer service

6. Choosing the right pharmacy system has been one of the tougher questions faced by pharmacies. However, successes in this area show that it is a critical decision that needs to be evaluated and planned for carefully with a 5-10 year roadmap in view. Given the multitude of considerations and individual operational nuances, the choice often is specific to each pharmacy chain.

SUMMARY:

Drugstore and pharmacy are the same but may be drugstores are not always required to have a pharmacist if they only sell medicine but not make them. In pharmacies can prepare prescription medicine. Adequate spaces, equipment and supplies are provided for the professional and administrative functions of the Pharmacy Service to assure patient safety through the proper storage, preparation (compounding, packaging and labeling) and dispensing of drugs.

A pharmacy needs to be designed to maximize the efficiency of the processes conducted to create the goods and services. The location of the pharmacy can affect: how easily and efficiently the inputs for operations can be acquired, how easily the outputs of operations can be transferred to the consumers of those outputs and which outputs are chosen to be offered by a given business (designing of goods and services).

Salesmanship is the process of applying three way management process (planning, implementation and evaluation) to sales force and its activities. Sales executive begin by setting sales goals and planning sales force activities.

Accounting records in drug stores will normally consists of cash/bank, receipts/payments, journal vouchers, etc. Various books of accounts, such as cashbook, bankbook and ledgers, can be generated and maintained using this module. It can also generate trial balance, balance sheet, and profit and loss statements.

REVIEW QUESTIONS

1. Discuss the different roles played by the pharmacist in a drug store?
2. How do you operate a drug store in a hospital?
3. Discuss the various issues involved in a community pharmacy and the role played by community pharmacist?
4. What are the different issues to be considered in pharmacy location?
5. Discuss the different layouts of a drug store? Explain the various advantages and disadvantages?
6. Explain the various principles followed in drug store administration?
7. What are the different guidelines for correct administration for medicines?
8. Define the term sales and discuss the concept of salesmanship?
9. What is sales promotion? Discuss in detail

GLOSSARY

B2B (Business-to-Business): Electronic communication and transactions among business entities such as manufacturers, retailers, and suppliers

B2C(Business-to-Consumer): Electronic communication and transactions between businesses and their customers.

Bulk Drug Manufacturers Association: was formed in 1991 with Hyderabad as its Head Quarters. The Association works for the consolidation of gains of the industry and serves as a catalyst between the government and the industry on the various issues for the growth of the industry

Business organisation: It is a process or an art of establish effective cooperation between the factors of production (land, material, capital equipment, personnel) for producing or acquiring wealth with a view to earn profit in an enterprise.

Buying: (Raw material to produce goods and services and to purchase finished goods or services as retailer or wholesaler to sell them again for final customers and consumers). It is a function that ensures that product offerings are available in sufficient quantities to meet customer demands.

CAD: Computer Aided Design is software which helps the designer to make the three-dimensional design of a product on the computer and visualize the design from various angles.

CAM: Computer Aided Manufacturing is a form of automation in which computers are used in process control, ranging from controlling various machines to controlling even the process quality.

Cellular Layout: A lay out that creates individual cells process parts or customers with similar requirements.

$\bar{x}$ **chart:** A control chart used to control the average of the process.

Clinical pharmacy care: direct health care and consultation provided by clinically trained pharmacists to patients and consumers about prescription and nonprescription drugs, and related products

Clinical pharmacy: pharmacy practice philosophy that has shifted the focus of pharmacists from drug products themselves to the safe and optimally effective use of drug products in patients; this philosophy positions pharmacists as active members of the health care team, working side by side with physicians and nurses, to provide direct care to patients and consultation to patients' families

Clinical trial: A research program conducted with patients to evaluate a new medical treatment, drug, or device the purpose of the clinical trial is to find new and improved methods of treating different diseases and special conditions.

Clinical trials: prospective studies in humans that compare the effectiveness and value of a potential new drug or therapy in one group against a control group before the drug or therapy is made available to the general population

Control chart: A graph containing three horizontal lines apart from the x-axis in which the top line is called as the upper control limit, the middle line is the central line and the bottom line is the lower control limit.

Decline: The period when sales show a downward drift and profits erode.

Drug delivery systems: methods of transporting drugs into the body or to specific sites of action in the body

Drug development: research process following drug discovery that takes a molecule with desired biological effects in animal models and prepares it as a drug that can be used in humans

Drug policy: any policy that affects the use and application of drugs, including legislative drug policies, insurance company drug policies, and hospital drug policies

Drug therapy management: management by pharmacists of the range of factors, such as drug dose, method of delivery, toxicity, and cost, that can affect the access to and effective use of drugs by patients

E-Commerce: Trade that occurs over a computer network, usually the Internet; more generally known as e-business

e-detailing is the use of the internet as the medium of communication for pharmaceutical sales detailing of physicians. It is a pharmaceutical or medical device firm-sponsored, internet-based program that informs prescribers about products or diseases using digital technology.

Element: It is a distinct part of a specified job selected for convenience of observation, measurement and analysis.

ERP: Enterprise Resource Planning is integration of enterprise wide information systems. Such system will link together all if a company's operations including human resources, financials, manufacturing and distribution as well as connect the organisation to its customers and suppliers.

Facility Layout: It is the arrangement of machines, departments, workstations and other areas with in a facility.

Facility: A facility could connote and physical object, be it a factory, hospital or Bank, relevant to location analysis.

Fixed-position layout: The product, because of its size and/or weight, remains in one location and processes are brought to it.

Flow process charts: A flow process chart is a process chart setting out the sequence of the flow of a product or a procedure by recording all activities under review using the appropriate process chart symbols. Flow process charts are of three types namely man, Material and Machine flow process chart.

FMS: Flexible Manufacturing System has a number of machines controlled simultaneously by a computer program in intermittent processes to process a variety of similar products. It is flexible to some extent, as the computer program can be modified to suit changes in processing requirements.

Food and Drug Administration: The FDA, an agency within the U.S. Public Health Service, which is a part of the Department of Health and Human Services.

Franchise: This is a special license from one organization to another to operate the business in great measure determined by the granting organization. For example, a licensee may own a motel that operates as a Holliday Inn.

Generic Drugs: A generic drug is identical, or bioequivalent to a brand name drug in dosage form, safety, strength, route of administration, quality, performance, characteristics and intended use. Although generic drugs are chemically identical to their branded counterparts, they are typically sold at substantial discounts from the branded price.

Generic: 1. The chemical name of a drug. 2. A term referring to the chemical makeup of a drug rather than to the advertised brand name under which the drug may be sold. 3.A term referring to any drug marketed under its chemical name without advertising.

Growth stage: A period of rapid market acceptance and substantial profit improvement.

Health care providers: health profes sionals, such as physicians, pharmacists, registered nurses, nurse practitioners, and dentists, who provide patient care

Health Insurance: is an insurance policy where the insurer assures the insured to compensate the loss incurred due to injury or illness. Health insurance offers compensation for medicine, hospitalizations, doctor visit and follows check ups and many other medical expenses

Insurance: is a mean to remove the hindrance of risk. risk factor is reduced by insurance. There are life insurance, fire insurance, marine insurance, car insurance, medical insurance and many more insurance facility given by insurance companies

Introduction Stage: A period of slow sales growth as the product is introduced n the market. Profit are nonexistent I this stage because of the heavy expenses incurred with product introduction.

JIT (Just-in-Time): Integrated activities designed to achieve high volume production using minimal inventories of raw materials, work-in-process, and finished products.

Joint Venture: This is a business combination of two or more companies that creates a third company to perform a specific function or to handle a specific business.

Life Insurances: are such kind of insurances that are paid to named beneficiaries when the insured person dies. Life insurance provides a monetary benefit to the family member or a relative to a decedent

Manufacturing: It is a process of converting raw material in to finished product by using various processes, machines and energy. It is a narrow term. Production is a process of converting inputs in to outputs.

Marine insurance: falls under commercial insurance. The policy is taken to reduce business risks. It caters to small scale business organisations to large corporates. Policy does not cover loss or damage due to willful misconduct, ordinary leakage, improper packing, delay, war, strike, riot and civil commotion.

Marketing: is a social and managerial process by which individuals and groups obtain what they need and want through creating and exchanging products and value with others.

Mass production: (also called flow production, repetitive flow production, series production, or serial production) is the production of large amounts of standardized products, including and especially on assembly lines.

Materials: The selection of materials for the product. Production manager must have sound knowledge of materials and their properties, so that he can select appropriate materials for his product. Research on materials is necessary to find alternatives to satisfy the changing needs of the design in the product and availability of material resumes.

Maturity: A period of slowdown in sales growth because the product has achieved acceptance by most potential buyers. Profits stabilize or decline because of increased competition.

Method study: It is the "systematic recording and critical examination of existing and proposed ways of doing work, as a means of developing and applying easier and more effective methods and reducing costs.

Methods: Finding the best method for the process, to search for the methods to suit the available resources, identifying the sequence of process are some of the activities of Production Management

Micromotion study: These studies are based on the concept of dividing human activity (body movements) into groups of movements called therbligs, according to the purpose for which they are made.

Motion Study: It is a type of method analysis at the micro level to determine the individual motions required to accomplish a task or a job.

New product development: NPD is the term used to describe the complete process of bringing a new product or service to market

Normal Time: It is the time required to perform an explicitly defined task at the agreed pace by an individual possessing the metal and physical ability.

Operations Management: Design, operation, and improvement of the systems that create and deliver the firm's primary products and services.

OTC: Over-the-counter products i.e. products sold without a prescription (OTC drugs, dietary supplements and other medicinal products)

Outline process chart: It gives a 'birds – eye' view of the entire activity by recording in sequence the main operations and inspections of a whole process or activity.

Pharmacy Council of India (PCI) The Pharmacy education and profession in India up to graduate level is regulated by the PCI, a statutory body governed by the provisions of the Pharmacy Act, 1948 passed by the Parliament

Pharmacy: A retail outlet where drugs are sold/given to patients; pharmacies usually sell Rx, OTC drugs, parapharmaceuticals such as dietary supplements, dermocosmetics, as well as dressing, toothpastes and medical devices; 2) a branch of medical and chemical sciences which deals with medications, their application, composition etc.

Physician "Detailing": Direct physician contacts by pharmaceutical manufacturers to instruct providers about their products in plans of influencing the physician's prescribing patterns

PMTS: A predetermined Motion Time System (PMTS) is a work measurement technique whereby times established for basic human motions (classified according to the nature of the motion and the conditions under which it is made) are used to build up the time for a job at a definite level of performance.

Process charts: These are the charts drawn to show how the material is processed from the raw material stage to the finished goods stage,

Process Layout: A layout that groups similar activities together into work centers according to the process or function they perform

Product layout: A layout that arranges activities in a line according to the sequence of operations that are needed to assemble a particular product.

Production management deals with decision-making related to production processes so that the resulting goods or service is produced according to specifications, in the amounts and by the schedule demanded and at minimum cost.

Production System: System by which resources are used to transform inputs into desired output.

Production: According to E.S. Buffa production is a process by which goods and services are created.

Productivity: It is defined as the ratio of output produced to the input resources utilised in the production.

Property insurance: gives protection against your property. This includes specialized forms of insurance like fire insurance, flood insurance, earthquake insurance, home insurance etc.

Qualified worker: A qualified worker is the one who is accepted as having the necessary physical attributes, who possesses the required intelligence and education, and who has acquired the necessary skill and knowledge to carry out the work in hand to satisfactory standards to safety, quality and quantity.

Quality : American society for quality defines it as "the totality of features and characteristics of a product or service that bases on its ability to satisfy stated or implied needs".

Quality Assurance : Quality assurance is defined as the system of policies, procedures and guidelines that establishes and maintains specified standards of product quality.

Quality Circles : 'Quality Circle' also called quality teams or quality task forces are as a unit is an integrated system constituting small groups of people (of about 8 to 10 persons) from same or similar work areas, who voluntarily offer to meet in order to identify, analyse and solve problems, which may lead to improvement in their total performance and enrichment of their work life.

Quality control : Bethel, Atwater and Stackman defines quality control as "the systematic control of those variables encountered in a manufacturing process which affect the excellence of the end product. Such variables result from the application of materials, men, machines and manufacturing conditions".

Quality control: refers to all those functions or activities that must be performed to fulfill the company's quality objectives. Hence, quality control involves the establishment of quality standards, the use of proper materials, the selection of appropriate manufacturing processes and the necessary tooling to make the product, the performance of the necessary manufacturing operations and finally the inspection of the product to check on the conformance with the specifications.

R chart: A control chart used to control the variability of the process.

Relaxation Allowances: Relaxation allowance is an addition to the basic time intended to provide the worker with the opportunity to recover from the physiological and pshychological effects of carrying out specified work under specified conditions and to allow attention to personal needs. The amount of allowance will depend on the nature of the job.

Retail Pharmacy Networks: Pharmacies with whom a Pharmacy Benefit Manager or insurance carrier has employed and contracted with, and with whom discounts are negotiated for drug ingredients and dispensing fees.

S Q C : S.Q.C is the application of quantitative techniques to determine how far the product conforms to the standards of quality and precision and to what extent its quality deviates from the standard quality.

Sales promotion: consists of diverse collection of incentive tools, mostly short term designed to stimulate quicker or greater purchase of particular product or services by consumers or the trade. Sales promotion is the process of persuading a potential customer to buy the product. It can be part of the personal selling process.

Selling: The function to be performed to sell the products/services/idea to satisfy customer needs or wants by using advertising, personal selling and sales promotion to match goods and services to customer needs.

Sole Proprietorships: A sole proprietorship is the easiest organization to form or to understand. Most small businesses are or were originally sole proprietorships. Essentially, any business not of any other form is a proprietorship. It is the form of business started out by anyone who just starts a business.

Specialty Drugs: Utilized by a small percentage of the population with rather complex and/ or chronic conditions (like MS, hepatitis C, rheumatoid arthritis, organ transplants) requiring costly and/or difficult drug regimens (like injectible and infusion therapies). Moreover, specialty drugs may need particular handling such as refrigeration

Specifications : Specifications are a detailed descriptions or listing of the characteristics of material parts and components used in making a product.

Standard Time: It is the time taken by a qualified worker for a specific task or Job, working under moderate conditions and including other allowances such as allowances for fatigue, setting of tools for job, repairing of tools etc.

Standard Time: It is the time taken by a qualified worker for a specific task or job, working under moderate conditions and including other allowances such as allowances for fatigue, setting of tools for job, repairing of tools etc.

Standards : Quality standards relate to time, materials, performance, reliability and appearance or any quantifiable characteristic of the product.

Strategic Alliance: In this case, two or more organizations agree to work together to accomplish a goal. For example, one company may manufacture a product but have poor marketing, so it forms a strategic alliance with a marketing company

Supply chain management: The supply chain is understood as a network of flows from initial suppliers to final recipients. This network covers flows in supplies, production, distribution and other flows related to customer service, operations regarding research, development, marketing etc. Supply chain management, if defined in this way, consists of the integration of key processes from supplier to final user in order to add value to products, services and information. SZP Spolocna Zdravotna Poistovna, Slovakia

Total work content: Basic work content + Excess time where basic work content is the irreducible minimum time theoretically required to produce one unit of output.

Transformation Process: Every process in an organisation, be it a product or service organisation, transforms certain inputs into outputs. This is called the transformation process.

Transporting: Function related to create the availability of product or services. It is used for moving products from their points of production to location convenient for purchases

Work Measurement: It is defined as the application of techniques designed to establish the time for a qualified worker to carry out a specific job at a defined level of performance.

Work Measurement: It is the "application of techniques designed to establish the time for a qualified worker to carry out a specified job at a defined level of performance.

Work Measurement: It is the "application of techniques designed to establish the time for a qualified worker to carry out a specified job at a defined level of performance."

Work Sampling: It is a method of finding the percentage occurance of a certain activity by statistical sampling and random observations.

Work Study: It is a generic term for those techniques, particularly method study and work measurement, which are used in the examination of human work in all its contexts, and which lead systematically tot he investigation of all the factors which affect the efficiency and economy of the situation being reviewed, in order to effect improvement.

REFERENCES

1. Adam E.E. and Ebert R. J., Production Operation Management, Fifth Edition, Prentice Hall of India Pvt. Ltd., New Delhi,

2. B V Patel Pharmaceutical Education and Research and Development (PERD) Centre, Ahmedabad and United Nations Industrial Development Organisation, New Delhi. ' *Diagnostic Study of Drugs and Pharmaceutical Clusters in Ahmedabad and Vadodara'*, August 2000.

3. Basant Rakesh, (1997), 'Analysing Technology Strategy Some Issues'. *Economic and Political Weekly*, 32(48), P: M111-120.

4. Bioscope, Sanfrancisco Chronicle, January 1, 2001.

5. Bowander. (1998), ' Industrialization and Economic Growth of India: Interactions of Indigenous and Foreign Technology', *International Journal of Technology Management*. 15(6,7), P622-645.

6. Buffa E. S. and Sarin R.K., Modern Production Operation Management, 8th Ed., John Wiley & Sons, 1987.

7. Centre for Monitoring Indian Economy (2000), Industry, Market Size and Shares, Mumbai, August.

8. Chary , S. N., Production and Operation Management, Tata McGraw Hill, New Delhi, 1988.

9. Chary,S.N. *Theory and problems in Production and Operations Management*, TMH Outline series, Nwedelhi

10. Chase, R.B., and N. J. Aquilano, Production and Operations Management: A Life Cycle Approach : 7th Ed., Irwin Inc.

11. Chaudhuri Sudip., (1999), 'Growth and Structural Changes in the Pharmaceutical Industry in India', in *The Structure of Indian Industry* (ed), Sen Anindya, Gokarn Subir and Vaidya Rajendra, Oxford University Press, New Delhi.

12. Correa Carlos M., (2000) *'Intellectual Property Rights, the WTO and Developing Countries: The TRIPS Agreement and Policy Options'*, Zed Books Ltd, London and Third World Network, Malaysia.

13. Danzon M Patricia and Chao Wei-Li.., (2000) 'Does Regulation Drive Out Competition in Pharmaceutical Markets?', *The Journal of Law and Economics,* 43(2) October.

14. Davis, Mark M., Aquilano, Nicholas J., & Chase, Richard B., Fundamentals of Operations Management (3rd.ed.) Irwin/ McGraw-Hill, Chicago, 1999.

15. Dilworth, James B. Operations management: providing value in goods and services. 3rd ed. Fort Worth: Dryden Press; 2000)

16. Donald Waters, Operations Management, Price Waterhouse Coopers, PricewaterhouseCoopers (Firm), PricewaterhouseCoopers LLP 1999

17. Dunning John (1992), *'Multinational Enterprises and the Global Economy'*, Addison-Wesley Publishers Ltd, UK.

18. Everett. Adam, Jr. and Ronald J. Ebert: Production and Operations Management, Concepts, Models and Behaviour, Pearson education,2003.

19. Express Pharma Pulse, Various Issues, Mumbai

20. Frank Richard and Salkever David. (1992), 'Pricing, Patent Loss and the Market for Pharmaceuticals', *Southern Economic Journal,* 59(2).

21. Gadbaw Michael and Richards Timothy., (1988), *'Intellectual Property Rights, Global Consensus, Global Conflict'* (ed) West view Press, London.

22. Gambardella Alfonso (1995), *Science and Innovation, The US Pharmaceutical Industry During the 1980s.* Cambridge University Press, New York.

23. *GATT Agreements-Final Text of Uruguay Round* (1994), MVIRDC, World Trade Centre, Bombay.

24. Government of India, (2000), Handbook of Industrial Policy and Statistics, New Delhi.

25. Grabowski Henry and Vernon M John. (1992), 'Brand Loyalty, Entry and Price Competition in Pharmaceuticals after the 1984 Drug Act', *Journal of Law and Economics,* 35(2), October.

26. Grabowski Henry. (1968), 'The Determinants of Industrial Research and Development: A Study of the Chemical, Drug and Petroleum Industries', *The Journal of Political Economy*, 76(2). March-April, P: 292-306.

27. Herman Christian Nolen, Harold Howard Maynard, " Drug Store Management", McGraw-Hill book company, inc., 1941

28. *Intellectual Property Rights,* (IPR) Various Issues, Patent Facilitating Centre, Department of Science and Technology, New Delhi.

29. International Intellectual Property Institute, (2000), *'Patent Protection and Access to HIV/AIDS Pharmaceuticals in Sub-Saharan Africa'*, Washington.

30. James B. Dilworth, Production and Operations Management : Manufacturing and Services, 5th Ed., Mc. Graw-Hill International.

31. Jensen J.E., (1987). 'Research Expenditures and the Discovery of New Drugs', *Journal of Industrial Economies*, 36(1).

32. K Ashwathappa and K Sridhara Bhat: Production and Operations Management, Himalaya Publishing House, 2002.

33. K S Menon: Purchasing and Material Control, Wheeler Publishing House,3rd edition.

34. K.Aswathappa and K.Shridhara Bhat, *Production and Operations management*, 1st Edn, Himalayan Publishing Hpouse, Mumbai, 2001.

35. Kanishka Bedi, Production and Operations Management, Oxford University Press, Chennai, 2004

36. Keayla B K (1994a), 'Patent Protection and the Pharmaceutical Industry', in Nair K R G and Ashok Kumar (ed), *'Intellectual Property Rights'*, Allied Publishers, New Delhi.

37. Kirim S Arman. (1985), 'Reconsidering Patents and Economic Development: A Case Study of the Turkish Pharmaceutical Industry', *World Development*, 13(2), P219-236.

38. Knod, Edward M and Schonberger, Richard J: Operations Management – meeting customers' demands, McGraw Hill international, 7th edition, 2001.

39. Kumar Nagesh. (1996), 'Intellectual Property Protection, Market Orientation and Location of Overseas R&D activities by Multinational Enterprises', *World Development*, 24(4), April, P673-688.

40. Lalitha N., (2001), ' *Product Patents and Pharmaceutical Industry'*, a report submitted to the Indian Council of Social Science Research, New Delhi.

41. Lanjouw Jean. (1998), *'The Introduction of Pharmaceutical Product Patents in India:" Heartless Exploitation of the Poor and Suffering?'* NBER Working Paper Series, Working Paper No.6366, National Bureau of Economic Research, Cambridge.

42. Lee J.Krajewski and Larry P.Ritzman, Operations Management – Strategy and Analysis, 6th Edn,Pearson Education, New Delhi, 2002

43. Madanmohan., (1997),'Exit Strategies: Experience of Indian Pharmaceutical Firms', *Economic and Political Weekly*, 32(48), P: M107-110.

44. Mahesh Burnade, D. "Principles and Practices of drug store Administration", Nirali Prakashan, 2008

45. Mansfield Edwin., (1986), 'Patents and Innovation: An Empirical Study', *Management Science*, 32(2), February, P173-181.

46. Martinich, Joseph S.: Production Operations Management- An Applier Modern Approach, JW, 2002.

47. Mehrotra., (1989), 'Patents Act and Technological Self-Reliance: The Indian Pharmaceutical Industry' *Economic and Political Weekly*, 24(19), P: 1059-1064.

48. Narayana, P.L. "The Indian pharmaceutical industry: problems and prospects, National Council of Applied Economic Research, 1984

49. Nogues Julio. (1990), *'Patents and Pharmaceutical Drugs: Understanding the Pressures on Developing Countries'*, Working Papers WPS 502, World Bank, Washington.

50. Ordover. (1991), 'A patent System for Both Diffusion and Exclusion', *Journal of Economic Perspectives*, 5(1), Winter, P43-59.

51. Panneerselvam,R., Production and Operations Management, Prentice Hall of India, New Delhi, 2002

52. Pannerselvam, R.: Production and operations Management, PHI,2002.

53. Pharmaceuticals: The Indian Pharmaceutical Industry, Feb 2005, ICRA

54. Philip Kotler, "Principles of Marketing, 2nd Edition, Prentice Hall international 2003

56. Philip Kotler, Kevin Lane Keller "Marketing Management", PHE,12/E, 2005

57. Pillai Mohanan. (1983) *'Policy Intervention and Response: A Study of the Pharmaceutical Industry in India During the Last Decade'*, CDS Working Paper No.218, Centre for Development Studies, Trivandrum.

58. Pillai, S.V. "The Indian pharmaceutical industry: a decade of achievements : speech", OPPI, 2007

59. Prasad Ashok Chandra and Bhat Shripad (1993), ' Strengthening India's Patent System, Implications for Pharmaceutical Sector' *Economic and Political Weekly*, 28(21), May, P.1037-1058.

60. Ramana Murthy, P. " Production and Operations Management", Revised Second edition, New Age International Publishers, 2007

61. Ramesh Govindraj, "The Indian Pharmaceutical Sector: issues and options for health sector", The world bank, 2002

62. Rane Wishwas (1995), 'Drug Prices: Sharp Rise after Decontrol', *Economic and Political Weekly*, 30(47). November 25, P.2977-2980.

64. Reddy Prasada and Sigurdson. (1997), 'Strategic Location of R&D and Emerging Patterns of Globalization: The Case of Astra Research Centre India', *International Journal of Technology Management*, 14(2,3, &4), P344-361.

65. Report of the Pharmaceutical Research and Development Committee, (1999), *Transforming India into a Knowledge Power*, Government of India, New Delhi.

66. Report on Currency and Finance, (1998-99), Reserve Bank of India, Mumbai.

67. Robert J. Bolger, Jude P. West, "Chain drug store management and operations", Cornell University, 1984

68. Roberta S.Russel and Bernard W.Taylor III, Operations Management 4th Edn, Pearson Education, New Delhi, 2004

69. S N Chary: Production and operations Management, Tata McGraw Hill, 2nd edition.

70. S. L. Kapoor, R. Mitra, "Herbal Drugs in Indian Pharmaceutical Industry", Economic Botany Information Service, National Botanical Research Institute, 1979

71. Sachin Itkar, "Pharmaceutical Management" Nirali Prakashan, 2008

72. Scherer F M and Watal Jayashree (2001), 'Post Trips Options for Access to Patented Medicines in Developing Countries', *CMH Working Paper Series*, World Health Organisation, Geneva, June.

73. Schroder, Roger G., Operations Management : Decision Making in the Operations Function, 2nd Ed. McGraw Hill Book Co., New York, 1985.

74. Scotchmer Suzanne. (1991), 'Standing on the Shoulders of Giants: Cumulative Research and the Patent Law', *Journal of Economic Perspectives*, 5(1), Winter, P29-41.

75. Scrip's Year Book, 2000, VOL.1 and 2, PJB Publications, UK 2000.

76. Sen Gupta Amit. (1996), '*Impact of Policy Changes on Drug Policy and Drug Use*', Paper prepared for the All India Drug Action Network, Voluntary Health Association of India and the National Campaign Committee for Drug Policy, Rational Drug Campaign Committee, New Delhi.

77. Sherwood Robert M., (1993), 'Why a Uniform Intellectual Property System Makes Sense for the World', in '*Global Dimensions of Intellectual Property Rights in Science and Technology*' edited by Wallerstein M, Mogee Mary and Schoen Roberta, National Academy Press, Washington D.C., P.68-87

78. Siebeck W, Evenson Robert, Lesser William and Braga Carlos Primo., (1990) *'Strengthening Protection of Intellectual Property in Developing Countries A Survey of the Literature'*, World Bank Discussion Papers, No.112, The World Bank, Washington D.C.

79. Singh Lakhwinder. (2001), ' Public Policy and Expenditure on R&D in Industry', *Economic and Political Weekly*, 36(31), August 4-10, P: 2920-2924.

80. Singh Pradeep, 'Strategic Options in Managing IPRs: The Case of Viagra' Saket Industrial Digest, August, 2001, P: 26-28.

81. Srinivasan S., (1999) ' How Many Aspirins a Rupee?' *Economic and Political Weekly*, 34(9), February, P514-518.

82. The Economic Times 'India Arrives at the WTO', 21 November 2001, P: 8.

83. The Economist, 'The Right to Good Ideas', June 23-29, 2001.

84. The Economist. *'The Pharmaceutical Industry'*, February 21, 1998.

85. Thomas E. Hendrick, Franklin G, "Production/Operation Managemetn", academy of Management, 1985

86. Times of India, *'Pharma Policy not to Exempt R&D Savvy Cos from DPCO'*, July 12, 2001.

87. United Nations Conference on Trade and Development, (1996) *'The TRIPS Agreement and Developing Countries'*, Geneva.

88. Watal Jayashree. (2001), *'Intellectual Property Rights in the WTO and Developing Countries'* Oxford University Press, New Delhi.

89. William J. Stevenson: Production Operations Management, McGraw –Hill , N.Delhi, 6th Edition1999.

90. Zilberman David, Cherisa Yarkin and Heiman Amir., 'Knowledge Management and the Economics of Agricultural Biotechnology', in Santaniello, Evenson .R, Zilberman and Carlson (ed), *Agriculture and Intellectual Property Rights*, CAB International 2000.